The Alzheimer's
Caregiving Puzzle

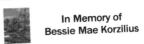

The Alzheimer's Caregiving Puzzle

Putting Together the Pieces

Patricia R. Callone, MA, MRE
Connie Kudlacek, BS

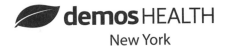

New York

Acquisitions Editor: Noreen Henson
Cover Design: Carlos Maldonado
Compositor: Newgen Imaging Systems
Printer: Bang Printing

Visit our website at www.demosmedpub.com

Medical information provided by Demos Health, in the absence of a visit with a healthcare professional, must be considered as an educational service only. This book is not designed to replace a physician's independent judgment about the appropriateness or risks of a procedure or therapy for a given patient. Our purpose is to provide you with information that will help you make your own healthcare decisions.

The information and opinions provided here are believed to be accurate and sound, based on the best judgment available to the authors, editors, and publisher, but readers who fail to consult appropriate health authorities assume the risk of any injuries. The publisher is not responsible for errors or omissions. The editors and publisher welcome any reader to report to the publisher any discrepancies or inaccuracies noticed.

Library of Congress Cataloging-in-Publication Data

The Azheimer's caregiving puzzle : putting together the pieces / Patricia R. Callone, Connie Kudlacek.
     p. cm.
   Includes index.
   ISBN 978-1-932603-88-0
   1. Alzheimer's disease—Popular works. 2. Caregivers. I. Callone, Patricia R.
II. Kudlacek, Connie.
   RC523.A36735 2011
   649.8084'6—dc22   2010030046

Special discounts on bulk quantities of Demos Health books are available to corporations, professional associations, pharmaceutical companies, health care organizations, and other qualifying groups. For details, please contact:

Special Sales Department

Demos Medical Publishing
11 W. 42nd Street
New York, NY 10036
Phone: 800–532–8663 or 212–683–0072
Fax: 212–941–7842
E-mail: rsantana@demosmedpub.com

Made in the United States of America

10 11 12 13   5 4 3 2 1

Contents

Preface

Why this book? Aren't there enough books on the market about Alzheimer's disease and caregiving? This is the third book we have published with Demos Health Publishing. Both of the other two books: *Alzheimer's Disease—The Dignity Within: A Handbook for Caregivers, Family and Friends* (2006) and *A Caregiver's Guide to Alzheimer's Disease: 300 Tips for Making Life Easier* (2006) continue to help caregivers of loved ones with Alzheimer's disease or other dementia.

However, through the growing body of knowledge about Alzheimer's disease and other dementia, we have developed new insights that need to be shared. From our own experiences, we have continued to learn more about "engaging" and "nurturing" persons with the disease as well as ways to "nurture" caregivers in the caregiving process. We continue to hear of ways in which persons with dementia can be exploited or abused. Family members and caregivers need to learn how to protect older persons who are most vulnerable in our society. We feel the "caregiving puzzle" of Alzheimer's disease—for both persons with the disease and their caregivers—needs to be revisited again.

We hope to plant new seeds for reflection about the dignified, appropriate, and safe care of persons with dementia and the appropriate care of caregivers.

Acknowledgments

We acknowledge the following people for their assistance in helping us shape the concepts and examples in this book.

Duane Gross, PhD, President and CEO, and Clayton Freeman, BA, Program Director, both from the Alzheimer's Association Midlands Chapter for their wealth of information and expertise they continue to share with us.

Noreen Henson, Director of Health Publications and Education, Demos Health, for her guidance and encouragement throughout the development of this book.

Helene L. Lohman, OTD, OTR/L, Associate Professor, Department of Occupational Therapy, School of Pharmacy and Health Professions, Creighton University. Helene teaches occupational therapy with elders. She is involved with the "Memories in the Making Project" through the Midlands Chapter of the Alzheimer's Association.

Patricia M. Sullivan, PhD, Professor of Psychiatry, School of Medicine, Creighton University. Dr. Sullivan is Co-Director of the Creighton Study of Violence Across the Lifespan and Director for The Center of Children's Issues. She has helped us understand the different ways in which vulnerable adults can be exploited or abused. Learning about those issues prompts caregivers to find ways to prevent abuse and exploitation of the most vulnerable among older adults—those with dementia.

Andrea Thinnes, OTD, OTR/L, Assistant Professor of Occupational Therapy and Director of Clinical Education, School of Pharmacy and Health Professions, Creighton University. Andrea is involved with the "Memories in the Making Project" through the Midlands Chapter of the Alzheimer's Association.

About the Authors

Patricia R. Callone, MA, MRE, met Connie Kudlacek in 1986 when her mother was diagnosed with Alzheimer's disease. She continues to be a volunteer with the Alzheimer's Association Midlands Chapter and has served as Vice President and President of the Board of Directors as well as on support committees concerning education and legislative issues. Pat has been a caregiver since she was 8 years old when her father was diagnosed with multiple sclerosis. She has cared for persons in her family who have had various illnesses including Alzheimer's disease. For 18 years, she was a caregiver to three people in her family who had dementia. She is involved in the community concerning aging issues and holds a leadership position in the Coalition to Protect Aging Adults (CPAA).

Connie Kudlacek, BS, was Executive Director of the Alzheimer's Association Midlands Chapter from 1986 to 2006. During that time, she met and worked with many committed and dedicated individuals who were caregivers to persons with Alzheimer's disease. Her personal caregiving experience has spanned over 55 years—beginning with caring for her mother who had cancer and continuing for the last 29 years as a caregiver to her son, who at the age of 18, experienced a severe closed head injury. She also continues to care for family relatives who have Alzheimer's disease and is actively involved in elder issues within her community.

In 2003, Connie and Pat formed a partnership and created *CaringConcepts, Inc.* (www.caringconcepts.org)

Contributors

Roger A. Brumback, MD, is a Professor of Pathology and Psychiatry and Chairman of the Department of Pathology, Creighton University School of Medicine, Omaha, Nebraska. He has been associated with the work of the Alzheimer's Association for many years. He and his wife, Mary, have served as long-distance caregivers to members in their families diagnosed with Alzheimer's disease.

Charles Timothy Dickel, EdD, is a longtime faculty member at Creighton University and currently holds the titles of Professor of Education, Professor of Psychiatry, and Co-Director of the Creighton Study of Violence Across the Life Span. In 1986, Tim was invited to form a support group of Alzheimer's family members by the local Alzheimer's Association. This began more than 20 years of interest in the well-being of caregivers and family members of persons diagnosed with dementia.

Juli-Ann Gasper, PhD, is Associate Professor, College of Business Administration, Creighton University, Omaha, Nebraska. She teaches finance classes that focus on social welfare, public policy with respect to vulnerable populations, and risk management for individuals, households, and non-financial businesses. She has more than 30 years of experience working with the elderly and seeking intellectual pursuits relating to financial issues of the elderly. She wrote one of the first dissertations (1984) about how widespread reverse mortgage availability could affect the financial well-being of elders. Juli-Ann was a caregiver to her father who had Alzheimer's disease.

Janaan Manternach, DMin, taught at Theological College and The Catholic University of America in Washington, DC; St. Mary's Seminary in Baltimore, Maryland; and St. Michael's College in Winooski, Vermont. Her passions include helping caregivers of individuals with Alzheimer's disease and homeless women and children, and writing children's literature and poetry. For many years, she was a caregiver to her husband, Carl Pfeifer, who had Alzheimer's disease.

Barbara Markey, ND, PhD, has been a marriage and family therapist for more than 30 years. Throughout that time, Barbara has worked with many caregivers. Dr. Markey completed her post-doctoral studies in family therapy at the Menninger Foundation. As a developmental psychologist and researcher, she has developed programs that emphasize growth and management of stresses over the life cycle. Recently, she was Associate Director of the Research Center for Marriage and Family at Creighton University, Omaha, Nebraska. She is an internationally recognized lecturer and trainer, and her family-related programs have been translated into many languages.

Lauren M. Petit, BA, Holy Cow! Word Processing. For many years, she has worked with older persons—including Holocaust survivors—to document their life experiences in written and digital formats.

Barbara Vasiloff, MA, is an educator and co-creator of "Discipline with Purpose—A Developmental Approach to Teaching Self-Discipline," a program used in more than 1,000 public and private schools in the United States. She is currently caring for both of her parents who are in their 90s. Her mother has dementia and her father is physically very frail. Barbara has put all of "The Discipline with Purpose" materials online so she can continue operating her business at her parents' home.

Introduction

According to the document "2009 Alzheimer's Disease Facts and Figures" developed by the National Alzheimer's Association, there are about 5.3 million people in the USA with Alzheimer's disease. It is estimated that about every 70 seconds someone is being diagnosed with the disease.

It is most common for Alzheimer's disease to be recognized in persons older than 65 years of age. We also know that the early onset of Alzheimer's disease (before 65) is becoming more apparent and that Alzheimer's disease seems to be increasing in the Black and Hispanic cultures. Statistics tell us that possibly one-out-of-two persons older than 85 years of age will have some dementia.

Additionally, about 10 million Americans provide unpaid care for persons living with Alzheimer's disease or other dementia. Families who have had someone diagnosed with Alzheimer's or other dementia live with the burden of knowing there is no cure at this time. But you probably know this. You are holding this book because, most likely, you are one of those people who have had Alzheimer's disease affect your family. You may be mourning the loss of the woman you once knew, or smiling when you catch just a glimpse of the man who raised you. Caring for a person with Alzheimer's disease is a difficult task and can become overwhelming at times.

Today, we hear that greater emphasis is being placed on how all of us can maintain the health of our bodies and brains through living healthy lifestyles—including diet, exercise, and attention to our environment. The hope is that practicing a healthy lifestyle will lead to less incidences of Alzheimer's disease. In addition to the focus on healthy life styles, we are seeing an emphasis on understanding the inner world of the person affected by Alzheimer's disease.

Scholars like Steven R. Sabat, Sam Fazio, and Dawn Brooker have focused on the "sense of self" bringing us new insights about the inner world of those affected by the disease. Sam Fazio states, "The self remains, however the ability to initiate it and maintain it is impaired because of the disease process." He also states that the self is influenced by other people, which is the most critical message for people who are providing dementia care.

This shift in focus to recognizing the person within or a "person-centered" concept is the main theme of the book, *Person-centered Dementia Care* by Dawn Brooker. This "person-centered" movement has partly been due to the fact that people with the disease have stepped forward and have given "voice" to the disease. It is a movement that is about building relationships between those who are caregivers and those who are cared for. This focus of education brings hope to those who believe that the "essence within" the person with Alzheimer's disease can be touched and empowered throughout the different stages of the disease. Throughout this journey, individuals are not to be recognized for their disease but for their individual uniqueness, which is created by their experiences, strengths, and interests.

As research continues into the study of the inner world and consciousness of persons with dementia, we, as caregivers, family members, and friends will have increased opportunities to explore new ways to live with those affected by the disease.

The authors of this book believe that caregivers, family members, and friends can enjoy the special skills, talents, joys, and humor of persons with dementia that remain intact throughout the progression of the disease. One example, which clearly shows how some functions continue to be accessible, is about the woman who had been in a nursing home for many years and had not spoken a word—only mumbling at times. When the woman was taken to church and the music would play, she would sing the hymns as if she had no dementia whatsoever. Another example is of a gentleman who spoke little and had an extremely short attention span, yet he could sit and play checkers by the hours at the adult day program.

Our goals are the following:

- Simplify the process/puzzle of Alzheimer's disease—the mind, the body, the self
- Expand the knowledge of the disease progression
- Propose unique concepts of care for persons experiencing dementia
- Support caregivers with information to keep them healthy in mind, body, and spirit
- Share personal and professional experiences of caregiving from nine caregivers

Caregivers and persons with dementia all need to understand these concepts in order to be involved with the issues discussed in the next pages. The underlying theme of all the chapters is "Nurture What Remains" of the mind, body, and spirit of persons with demen tia throughout the disease process.

Nurture What Remains

This phrase can sound a little dire, but really, it is a celebration. It is a conscious effort to engage persons with dementia who have been considered lost in the past, but whom we have come to realize are still there. To "Nurture What Remains" means to continue to grow and develop all parts of the mind, body, and spirit throughout life. It is up to all of us as caregivers to be "detectives" in the search for what will best socialize, stimulate, and keep the individual himself/ herself safe in the person's rhythms of each day.

Even though the progression of Alzheimer's disease brings loss, the "enduring self" remains and deserves continued nourishment. La Doris "Sam" Heinly wrote, "Through their art and their few remaining words, individuals with dementia tell us that they are still here, only in a unique way." Our challenge is to be able to tap into and engage that "enduring self" and offer opportunities to our loved ones to succeed in whatever capacity the person may have at that moment.

In her book, *Dancing with Dementia*, Christine Bryden wrote, "I believe that people with dementia are making an important journey from cognition, through emotions, into spirit. I've begun to realize what really remains throughout this journey is what is really impor-tant, and what disappears is what is not important. I think that if society could appreciate this, then people with dementia would be respected and treasured."

Today society deals with many attitudes about aging and dementia. It is easy to forget, or we may fail to acknowledge, that persons with Alzheimer's disease have the capacity to self-reflect and want to have a sense of purpose in the family or society. We must find ways to empower individuals to continue to be productive, to cope, to compensate for losses, and to adapt to their ever-changing lifestyles. In doing this for caregivers and individuals with dementia, we are recognizing everyone's value and dignity while living with Alzheimer's disease. The act of focusing on the remaining functions and individual spirit is the act of nurturing what remains.

This book has two parts. One addresses the care of persons with Alzheimer's disease and the other covers the care of caregivers, themselves. As we said before, we all know *Alzheimer's* care is a tough job. We aim, through this book, to make it just a little bit easier. Both parts of the book point out clues and cues that will help persons with Alzheimer's disease, other dementia, and their caregivers live meaningful lives, all the time concentrating on "What Remains," rather than what is lost.

The charts and grafts included in the text have been developed to illustrate the key functions that are controlled by the brain. They highlight what can be experienced at different stages of the disease process and can demonstrate how caregivers and persons with the disease can increase their understanding of the preserved functions that remain. When caregivers can increase their understanding of what is happening to the person who has the disease, they can more easily practice the concept of "Nurture What Remains."

The Alzheimer's journey presents many choices about living life. We are presented with the choice to improve our lives or we can live unbearable lives. As caregivers, we need to learn to live in the present. Seeing our loved ones in new ways helps us leave behind old habits and behaviors that may limit our ability to embrace persons with Alzheimer's disease with whom we are now living. It is time to develop a new relationship—a "caregiving partnership"—with our loved one. We have written this book—that contains personal and professional stories and advice from nine caregivers (authors)—to be a helpful companion to you in your caregiving days.

The Person with Alzheimer's Disease: One Piece of the Puzzle

CHAPTER 1

The Basics of Alzheimer's Disease and Dementia

Roger A. Brumback

As a caregiver to a loved one with Alzheimer's disease, it is important for you to understand the sometimes confusing terminology used by healthcare professionals, scientists, and even by the public to describe the disorder. It is most helpful to differentiate the terms "senility" and "dementia," which are often incorrectly equated with Alzheimer's disease. The term "dementia" means *the continuing loss of intellectual, cognitive, and thinking abilities sufficient to impair the ability to function day-to-day.* Thus, dementia is what you as a caregiver will notice about your loved one. You will notice memory problems, confusion, or difficulty performing ordinary tasks.

Dementia is what physicians call a "symptom." A symptom is not itself a disease. Rather it indicates the need to identify the cause of the disease. For example, a fever is a "symptom" that tells us something is causing a fever and the cause needs to be found. Dementia is a "symptom" that indicates something is wrong with the brain.

On the other hand, "senility" is not a medical term. Actually, prior to the 19th century, elderly individuals were usually revered for their wisdom and knowledge, and there are many examples of outstanding accomplishments by elderly individuals such as Michelangelo working on the design of St. Peter's Basilica up to his death at age 89 years; Titian painting masterpieces in Venice until his death at age 91 years; and Giuseppe Verdi (the foremost Italian opera composer) completing his masterpieces after age 70 years.

However, in order to halt calls for a revolutionary socialist agenda during the 1880s, the German Chancellor Otto von Bismarck established social welfare laws that mandated retirement at age 70 years (later lowered to 65 years). This was done because it was thought

3

people at that age would be less able to comprehend and live life. Thus, by legal decree, mental incompetence became viewed as part of the normal aging process. Today we know that this is not true and there are many current examples of persons living into their 90s and 100s who are living life well.

During this same period of the 19th century, European (particularly German) investigators were making major discoveries concerning the mechanisms of disease, and neuropsychiatrists were particularly interested in identifying brain changes. During microscopic brain studies of elderly individuals, Emil Redlick found peculiarly staining plaques (termed "senile plaques") that he thought explained senility. Alois Alzheimer confirmed those findings and subsequently reported the case of a 51-year-old woman who had shown memory loss, which progressed over the fourth year of a 5-year period to apathy, mutism, incontinence, and death. Alzheimer noticed the same kind of plaques (along with another feature called tangles) in her brain and hypothesized that she had an illness similar to the expected (and legislated) elderly senility.

The name Alzheimer's disease then came to designate a dementing illness occurring at an age younger than 65 years for the expected normal development of senility. The idea persisted through much of the 20th century that Alzheimer's disease was an uncommon disorder producing dementia as a result of a premature aging process. Only with the discoveries in the last decade of the 20th century have these ideas about senility as a normal aging process been abandoned.

It is now apparent that dementia is the result of many different conditions, which can interfere with the ability of the brain to work normally. In fact, for every 100 individuals seeking help from a primary care physician for the symptom of dementia, fully half of these individuals will have a treatable medical condition that is causing the symptom of dementia (Figure 1.1). (Physicians term this problem as "treatable dementia" or "reversible dementia.")

Examples of "treatable dementia" are the following:

Affective disorder (depressive pseudodementia)—Depression and bipolar disorder can produce memory and thinking disturbances.

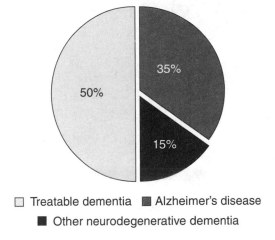

□ Treatable dementia   ■ Alzheimer's disease
■ Other neurodegenerative dementia

Figure 1.1   Treatable dementia or reversible dementia.

Multiple sclerosis—Cognitive and thinking problems are common in this autoimmune disease of the brain.

Drug- or medication-induced mental disturbances—Medications of all kinds can disturb thinking, particularly in older individuals; doses of ordinary medicines that have no effect in younger individuals can produce significant cognitive changes in elderly individuals.

Electrolyte imbalance; hypoglycemia—Changes in levels of the normal chemicals in the blood stream can affect thinking and memory.

Endocrine disorders (hypo- or hyperthyroidism, hypo- or hyperparathyroidism)—Hormones are important for normal brain function and altered levels can impair thinking and memory.

Epilepsy—Seizures impair memory.

Primary or secondary tumors—Brain tumors put pressure on the brain and impact thinking and memory.

Neurosyphilis, HIV infection (AIDS)—Both syphilis and HIV destroy nerve cells in the brain.

Normal pressure hydrocephalus—Enlargement of the ventricles (fluid sacs within the brain) damage surrounding brain and impair thinking and memory.

Pulmonary lung disease with chronic hypoxia and/or hypercarbia—Low oxygen or high levels of carbon dioxide in the blood damage or destroy nerve cells.

Kidney or liver failure—The kidneys and liver normally filter poisonous substances out of the blood stream; build-up of these poisons can destroy nerve cells.

Toxin exposure (alcohol, lead, arsenic, mercury, manganese, organic toxins)—Various poisons (toxins) can slowly destroy nerve cells.

Trauma: subdural hematoma and others—Hemorrhages inside the skull can compress the brain and interfere with thinking and memory.

Vitamin deficiencies (B12, folate, niacin, thiamine)—Vitamins are critical for brain cells to function, and vitamin deficiencies can cause nerve cell death.

As a caregiver of a person diagnosed or suspected to have Alzheimer's disease or other dementia, you need to consult medical professionals about the changes you are seeing in your loved one. Identifying and potentially treating underlying medical problems is an important first step in evaluating the individual with dementia. However, if there are no identifiable medical problems, it is likely that the individual has a disease that is slowly destroying the brain. Physicians term such conditions as "neurodegenerative dementias" (disease causing the nerve cells to die). The various neurodegenerative dementias have surprisingly similar features even though each has a unique and distinctive abnormal protein substance deposited in the brain causing the nerve cells to stop functioning and die.

The most common neurodegenerative dementia is Alzheimer's disease, followed in frequency by frontotemporal dementia, also called Pick's disease, and diffuses Lewy body disease. Occasionally, individuals will actually have a combination of Alzheimer's disease and one of the other two conditions. Multiple strokes can also cause dementia, but this is actually rare; most individuals with strokes and dementia actually have neurodegenerative dementia such as Alzheimer's disease and the strokes just make the problem worse.

With an overall understanding of the terminology concerning dementia, you, as a caregiver for your loved one, will be able to understand the relationship of the clinical features of the dementia and the underlying destructive process that occurs in the brain.

Unfortunately, because the brain destruction cannot be seen, Alzheimer's disease and the other neurodegenerative dementias are really hidden problems. Contrast this with, say, a broken leg. Everyone can see the cast and knows how to accommodate the person with that broken leg. No caregiver would think of accusing the person with a broken leg of "faking it" or "just being uncooperative" for not participating or performing some activity. However, since Alzheimer's disease affects only the brain and is therefore hidden from the caregiver's view, it is common for caregivers to be very upset about the affected person's behavior.

By understanding how the disease affects the brain, you can appreciate why your loved one acts as he or she does and you can then provide proper assistance and accommodation. This is particularly important for you to know, since the disease affects different parts of the brain at different times, while unaffected parts of the brain continue to function. To go back to the analogy of the broken leg—the person with a broken leg would still be able to use arms and hands to feed himself or herself and be able to write or use a computer—since only the leg is injured while the other three limbs are okay.

Similarly, in the middle stages of Alzheimer's disease, your loved one will not be able to remember names or faces or current events but he/she can still use other parts of the brain. Your loved one might be able to beat family members in a game of dominos. (This is part of a true case history. Unfortunately, until the family members came to understand the brain changes, they were very angry at the man, for they had been attributing his behavior to meanness and stubbornness.)

To understand the effect of the brain destruction in neurodegenerative dementias, it is necessary to know a little bit about the normal brain. Although the brain weighs only about 3 pounds and could comfortably be held in the palm of the hand, it is the most important organ of the body. It is entirely different from other organs in that every nerve cell in the brain does something unique which only that nerve cell can do and no other nerve cell can do. This is in contrast, for example, to the liver, where the left half of the liver does the same as the right half of the liver and every liver cell does the same as every other liver cell. The same is true for the kidneys. The left kidney does the same as the right kidney, and a person can even lose one kidney because the remaining kidney takes over and does everything. In the brain, each part has a specific and unique function and all the parts must work together for the brain to perform properly. Loss of or damage to any part of the brain results in loss of that function since no other part of the brain can take over or carry on that function (Figure 1.2).

The portion of the brain that is involved in thinking is the wrinkled part that sits on top. Other books will have more specific diagrams of the whole brain, but we do not need them here. The cerebrum has an almost spherical shape and is divided in the center, so each half is termed a cerebral hemisphere: a right cerebral hemisphere and a left cerebral hemisphere. The thin surface layer of the cerebral hemispheres contains all the nerve cells and is called the cerebral cortex.

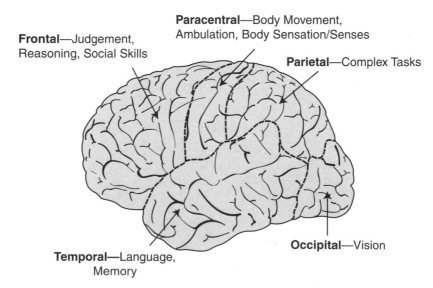

Figure 1.2   The brain hemispheres.

The cerebral hemispheres are subdivided into different lobes, which perform different specific functions. Refer to the brain diagram given earlier.

A strip of brain called the sensorimotor lobe is the part of the brain that initiates all body movements and feels all body sensations. It is divided in half, with the front half being motor area and the back half being sensory area. The motor area generates all body movement, but does so in a cross-over manner; that is, the motor area of the left cerebral hemisphere moves the right side of the body, while the right motor area moves the left side of the body. Similarly, the left sensory area feels the right side of the body and the right sensory area feels the left side of the body.

The back part of the cerebral hemispheres, called the occipital lobe, is for vision. The information from our eyes is developed into images in the visual area of the occipital lobes.

On the lower side of each cerebral hemisphere is the temporal lobe, which interprets the sound heard by our ears including language. For humans, there are two important qualities of sounds: speech sounds (language) and non-speech sounds (music, noises, and the tone and melody of speech). The temporal lobes contain "dictionaries" for interpreting all these sounds.

The parietal lobe is the area on the side of the brain situated between the visual (occipital), sound (temporal), and sensory areas of the brain. This part of the brain integrates together information from vision, hearing, and body sensation about our environment. For example, when reaching into a pant's pocket to get change, the coins will have a certain feel and sound as they clink together. The parietal lobe integrates this sensation information from the sensory area and the sound information from the temporal lobe to provide instructions to the hand to pick out the correct coins from other objects, such as keys, in the pocket. Then, when the handful of coins is brought out of the pocket and displayed, the parietal lobe integrates the visual information to confirm that the desired coins were correctly removed from the pocket.

The largest part of the brain is in front and is called the frontal lobe. This is the most "human" part of the brain and differentiates humans from lower primates and other animals. The frontal lobe is responsible for reasoning, judgment, logic, insight/foresight, self-awareness, and the control of the rest of the brain. This is sometimes called "executive control function." It contains all the rules of behavior that allow us to interact and live together in a society, including our ability to know right from wrong and what is socially acceptable or unacceptable.

In the lower center of the brain (on each side) is an area called the hippocampus (limbic lobe), which is responsible for cataloging and indexing all of our memories. As you can see, the brain is a very complex organ of the body. How it works and why it works the way it does is still being studied around the world. There is no cure for Alzheimer's disease today, but science continues to study the brain and all its mysteries to find a cure for dementias in general and Alzheimer's disease in particular.

All the neurodegenerative dementias cause the progressive death of nerve cells in the cerebral hemispheres of the brain, but nerve cells do not die all at once. Instead, there is a slow death march that moves from one area of the brain to the next area. Each of the disorders has a slightly different pattern to cell death.

It is important for you and your family to remember that while the destruction of some brain areas is occurring, other unaffected areas of the brain continue to function normally. The theme of "Nurture What Remains" needs to be applied throughout the disease process. Even though your loved one experiences the loss of some functions over a number of years, other functions will remain and should be stimulated and nurtured. Every person experiences dementia in different ways—according to the unique person he or she is.

Much of the literature about Alzheimer's disease suggests different stages of the disease. In this book, we speak about three stages of the disease to more clearly understand the progression of the disease: the Early-to-Mild Stage, the Moderate Stage, and the Severe Stage.

Early-to-Mild Stage: For the most common of these neurodegenerative dementias, Alzheimer's disease, the initial brain area in which nerve cells die is the hippocampus, which controls memory; thus, the first features of Alzheimer's disease are related to memory loss. However, since the rest of the brain functions well, the person still moves and feels things (controlled by the sensorimotor lobe), still sees (controlled by the occipital lobe), still hears (controlled by the temporal lobe), and still integrates information (controlled by the parietal lobe). Because judgment, reasoning, and social skills (controlled by the frontal lobe) are still functioning normally, the person can develop compensatory coping strategies to deal with the memory problems, like making lists or relying on others to remember.

With these compensations in this beginning stage of Alzheimer's disease process, the person will appear normal and not consult a physician, and the family members and friends will be unaware of any problems. Nonetheless, extensive and very careful neuropsychological testing can demonstrate the memory loss, which has been called "benign senile forgetfulness" or "mild cognitive impairment."

As the nerve cell destruction of Alzheimer's disease continues, the damage spreads out over the brain like a wave of destruction. When the temporal lobe is affected, the person will experience trouble understanding words or expressing correct words, causing conflicts with others or prompting the person to withdraw and communicate less. Again, since the remainder of the brain is still able to function normally, individuals with Alzheimer's disease rarely come to medical attention at this stage and the families do not obtain information about this caregiving solution. In this Early-to-Mild Stage (the auditory stage) of Alzheimer's disease, misunderstandings and suspicion arise because of the problems in communication. An example could help to illustrate this problem:

An elderly husband and wife are sitting at the breakfast table as they do every morning, and as the man is about to drink his coffee, he asks his wife to "pass the salt." She obliges and he becomes angry. What he actually wanted was the sugar to put in his coffee, but because of the Alzheimer's disease damage to his temporal lobe, the word came out as "salt." He is angry, because his wife has recently been responding to his requests like this every day. Since his frontal lobe judgment and reasoning are still intact, he has been trying to figure out why she is doing this and seems to have the answer: she knows he has high blood pressure and if he takes in more salt he will die and she can collect the life insurance. This is making him more suspicious of everything his wife does. At the same time, the wife is becoming increasing unhappy that her husband is so irritable when she does exactly what he asks her to do. The solution would be for the wife to recognize that her husband is having problems using the correct words, to anticipate his requests, and to respond appropriately (i.e., passing the sugar to him even though he says "salt").

Moderate Stage: In the moderate stage (parietal lobe stage) of Alzheimer's disease, the wave of nerve cell destruction spreads out over the parietal lobes, causing the person to lose the ability to integrate information from visual, sound (auditory), and body sensation cues. This is the stage at which the person experiences trouble dressing, getting lost or is disoriented, seems clumsy, and cannot figure out how to use objects.

For example, in the Moderate Stage, the person could just sit at a dinner table, but not be able to start eating because the visual information about food and utensils cannot be integrated. The person could well be hungry, but is unable to eat because of the language difficulties remaining from the previous stage of the illness. Your loved one will be unable to communicate the problem. You, as the caregiver, need to gently assist your loved one by placing the utensils in the correct hand, allowing him/her to experience the body sensation of the utensil in his/her hand. Your assistance will be enough for him or her to begin eating. In the previous situation, you need to recognize that your loved one generally will have difficulty asking for things or for help because the disease process has already passed through and devastated the temporal lobe speech areas.

In the Moderate Stage, the person gets lost. This is also the stage of the disease in which driving becomes problematic, because he/she cannot integrate all the visual and sound information of the environment with the proper body sensation of the steering wheel and floor pedals. The person can often compensate through strategies devised by using the still intact frontal lobes. Your loved one can still figure out ways to adapt to his/her environment. Persons with dementia are naturally using all the coping mechanisms they can to live in the environment that is changing for them.

At some point in this Moderate Stage of the progression of Alzheimer's disease, family members or friends usually recognize that a problem exists and encourages the person to consult physicians for evaluation and treatment. Generally, someone in the family takes the initiative to make an appointment with the doctor. Your loved one will not be able to or want to take the initiative to make the appointment.

Severe Stage: After devastating the parietal lobes, the Alzheimer's disease process moves into the frontal lobes, affecting the person's ability to interact properly with those around him or her. It is in this

Severe Stage (frontal lobe stage) that caregivers experience considerable problems providing care. The loss of judgment, reasoning, and social skills during this stage can result in inappropriate and socially unacceptable behaviors. For example:

> *In the moderate (parietal lobe) stage of Alzheimer's disease, the person could go out to a restaurant with family members, sit quietly, eat the meal with some help from family members with the utensils and the food, and behave appropriately for such a social situation. They may not, however, remember having eaten after the meal was over. However, during the frontal lobe stage of the disease, such a restaurant visit could be problematic because of the loss of judgment and normal social inhibitions could result in the person feeling warm and just stripping off all clothes to feel cooler.*

At varying times in the Severe Stage, with the loss of a sense of appropriate behavior because of the disease's impact on the frontal lobes, the person can become apathetic and immobile or possibly strike out at others. For example, touching (such as helping the person undress) can trigger a combative response—possibly injuring either the caregiver or the person with Alzheimer's disease. Episodes like the examples can become less when caregivers understand what is happening to the person and give him/her proper, dignified care. Part of the responsibility of caregivers is to find what is happening so both the caregiver and the person with dementia can live dignified lives.

Near the end, the destructive Alzheimer's disease process has severely damaged most of the brain's nerve cells. Nearly all the nerve cells of the cerebral hemispheres—except a strip of motor cortex and the visual cortex—have been damaged. This is why in nursing homes, the main activity seems to be walking and pacing. Finally, however, even these brain areas are destroyed and the individual will be bedridden and relatively unresponsive.

With frontotemporal dementia/Pick's disease the destructive wave across the brain takes a very different course. The initial destruction involves the frontal lobe causing the person in the Early Stage (frontal stage) of frontotemporal dementia to show behavioral problems. These problems are somewhat similar to those described in the Severe Stage of Alzheimer's disease. Since the rest of the brain still functions normally, the poor judgment and aberrant behaviors can be quite dangerous to family members and friends as well as to the person him- or herself.

Because these behavior issues seemingly appear "out of nowhere," family and friends will raise concerns about a possible "psychiatric disease" and push for an evaluation. Unfortunately, it is sometimes difficult to find mental health practitioners familiar with differentiating frontotemporal dementia from psychiatric conditions. However, the correct diagnosis becomes clear as the nerve cell destruction of frontotemporal dementia progresses to involve the parietal lobe in the Moderate Stage (parietal lobe stage). The person with the disease then shows evidence of clumsiness and disorientation. During the Severe Stage of frontotemporal dementia when the temporal lobes are destroyed, the individual will become noncommunicative. Interestingly, memory problems only are evident at the very end of the disease process.

Although generally resembling Alzheimer's disease, the course of diffuse Lewy body disease has less distinctive stages and sometimes resembles a mixture of Alzheimer's disease and frontotemporal dementia. It is therefore crucial for you, as a caregiver, and your family to have your loved one properly diagnosed. You, your family, and your loved one's friends can help the person with dementia to live the best possible life. You can develop strategies to accommodate lost functions and, more importantly, enhance the remaining abilities. . . . "Nurturing What Remains."

Throughout life, healthy areas of our brains are constantly changing based upon our experiences and education. A nerve cell connects with other nerve cells through its vast array of processes called dendrites. These dendrites resemble the branches of trees with the areas of interconnection resembling the leaves of the tree. As humans age, like the maturing of a tree, the nerve cells develop a complex and continuously enlarging canopy of dendritic processes through learning and experience. When an area of the brain is damaged, the nerve cells in surrounding healthy areas are triggered to greatly expand their canopy in an attempt to compensate for the loss. This is important in caregiving, since the person can be helped to utilize and enhance remaining abilities, while healthy nerve cells attempt to enlarge their scope of influence and compensate for the lost nerve cells.

CHAPTER 2

Stages of Alzheimer's Disease Defined

Connie Kudlacek

We have found it helpful to divide the progression of Alzheimer's disease into stages, as it can serve as a strategy for the evaluation and understanding of the preserved functions. There are several different perspectives on the number of stages used. We have chosen to simplify this concept and use only three stages to identify the disease process: the Early-to-Mild Stage, the Moderate Stage, and the Severe Stage. We also have added the Pre-Alzheimer's Disease Stage for clarification.

PRE-ALZHEIMER'S DISEASE STAGE

Frequently, we find that the Pre-Alzheimer's Disease Stage is commonly left off most lists as it is often seen traditionally as a stage of normalcy. This is why we do not list it in the stages of the disease process. However, we define and identify it because it gives us a basis from which to draw conclusions as we discuss the other three stages.

We know that a person's brain weighs only about 3 pounds and yet it is the most important part of the body. When a person's brain is healthy and has been kept active, all parts of the brain work together to allow the individual access to key brain functions. In the books *The Mature Mind: The Positive Power of the Aging Brain* and *The Creative Age: Awakening Human Potential in the Second Half of Life* by Dr. Gene D. Cohen, MD, PhD, it is stated that the brain grows, develops, and compensates to help perform tasks throughout life.

Also, Dr. Cohen reminds us that there is new knowledge about the brain that includes:

- The brain is continually resculpting itself in response to experience and learning.
- New brain cells do form throughout life.
- Studies demonstrate that exercise stimulates the production of important chemicals that increase brain cell activity.
- There are different types of memory, which are used throughout life.

We all develop differently and uniquely... according to our unique creation. The key point here is that we know now that the brain grows and develops throughout life.

The brain drawings and circle diagrams given in this chapter illustrate key functions that are controlled by the brain (Figure 2.1). How well a person is able to do each of these functions is based on innate abilities, education, training and practice, and a person's mental and physical health.

As indicated in the pie chart, we have divided each function equally. But we know that it is the rare individual who has developed each of these functions to the fullest potential. But even the modest ability of a person to perform each of these functions demonstrates that the nerve cells in the brain are healthy and working. This healthy brain can recall long-term and short-term memories. At times, memory cues can be used to recall, and can often help to cause both pleasant and unpleasant memories.

The functions are as follows:

Memory

When a person's brain is healthy and has been kept active, long-term and short-term memories can be recalled through concentration and focus. Memory cues can help trigger those memories. Some of those cues include sight, smell, taste, sound, sensations, people, and places. Each of us experience situations where we have occasional lapses of memory such as misplacing an item or forgetting someone's name. These types of memory lapses are normal and usually happen to most people as they get older.

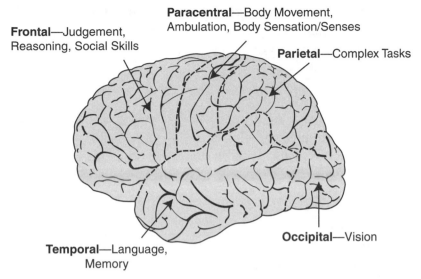

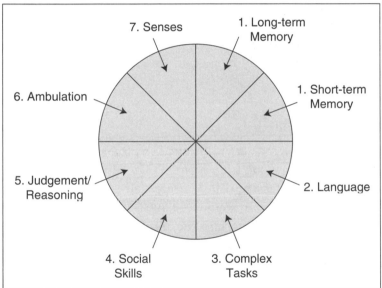

Figure 2.1   Brain functions and Pre-Alzheimer's disease. (Shaded areas show what functions remain).

Language

When a person's brain is healthy, a person is able to understand sounds, engage in the complex task of communicating effectively, and active listening. Forgetting what you were going to say or a person's name when the person has just introduced himself or herself can happen to anyone during his/her daily activities. This is not necessarily a sign of dementia.

Complex Tasks

These tasks are made up of many interrelated parts. Every day we use useful techniques to help us develop the skills necessary for completing many tasks, even at the same time. An example of a complex task would be to be able to balance a check book or follow an intricate recipe.

Social Skills

Research today continues to point out that social interaction is necessary in our lives and that social skills remain the glue that keeps people civilized and learning to appreciate diversity. A healthy person reaches out to others and allows them to respond. They also will interact appropriately in person, in written communications, via phone or Internet.

Judgment and Reasoning

During the late teenage years to the mid-twenties, a person's reasoning and judgment become fully formed. This enables the person to examine, organize, classify, differentiate, self-regulate, and self-correct among other things. Individuals have the ability to self-regulate and self-correct in situations, and the ability to differentiate and prioritize. To self-regulate would be to behave in an appropriate common manner rather than to give into impulses that result in socially unacceptable behaviors.

Ambulation

Moving, exercising, walking, running, swimming, and so on are important parts of life. They not only keep the person healthy but stimulate the brain as well. Ambulation is the ability to move from one place to another independently while walking, swimming, running, and so on.

Senses

The senses not only include sights, sounds, smell but also the acts of sharing, creating art, appreciating good food, and many other activities that enhance our quality of life. Individuals have the ability to create and appreciate pleasant surrounds or activities that bring satisfaction to their individual senses such as listening to music, enjoying good food, or sharing intimately with others.

When we observe continual decreases in key functions of the brain, it is only natural to wonder if it is a sign of old age or if that the brain is becoming diseased. However, characteristics of the normal aging process are that general intelligence remains normal and reasoning abilities and judgments are not altered. It may take longer to learn new skills, grasp new ideas, react to things, recall the right word or someone's name, but symptoms of Alzheimer's disease are actually much more problematic.

WHAT IS THE EARLY-TO-MILD STAGE?

In people with Alzheimer's disease, changes in the brain may occur 10 to 20 years before any visible signs or symptoms appear. Early in the disease process regions of the brain may begin to shrink, causing nerve cells to die off. This initial decline results in shrinkage in the memory area of the brain. In Dr. Brumback's material, we learned that symptoms of Alzheimer's disease are actually much more problematic than just the simple lapses in memory, and these symptoms begin to interfere with the ability to perform normal daily activities. Nevertheless, the person will learn ways to compensate for the failings until too many appear. Because judgment, reasoning, and social skills are still functioning normally, the person can develop compensatory coping strategies to deal with the memory problems.

Thus, as previously stated, in the beginning stage of the disease process, in most situations, these losses are not evident to others because of these compensations and the person will appear normal and often never consult a physician. Individuals with early symptoms often seem healthy, but they are actually having trouble understanding the world around them. It often takes time for observers to realize that something is wrong because the initial symptoms of Alzheimer's disease can often be confused with normal aging changes. The importance of early diagnosis though is that early intervention and treatment of Alzheimer's disease may delay the progression of the disease.

In the pie chart of the Early-to-Mild Stage, it shows the areas first affected by the disease process (Figure 2.2). The main areas affected are short-term memory and language skills with the other functions left intact.

EARLY-TO-MILD STAGE CLUES

A combination of some of these clues would describe a person who is "not as capable as he/she used to be." In this stage, a few of the following symptoms, taken from "The 10 Warning Signs of Alzheimer's Disease" (National Alzheimer's Association), will be occurring.

1. Memory changes that disrupt daily life
2. Challenges in planning or solving problems
3. Difficulty in completing familiar tasks
4. Has difficulty learning new things or making new memories
5. Confusion with time or space
6. Trouble understanding visual images and special relationships
7. New problems with words in speaking or writing
8. Losing the ability to retrace steps
9. Decreased or poor judgment
10. Depression symptoms (sadness, decreased energy and interest in usual activities)

Your loved one will need time for socialization and stimulation in an environment that is safe. He/she should also have access to the following:

• Knowledge about Alzheimer's disease or related dementia so that the person does not blame himself/ herself for what is occurring
• The assistance of family/caregivers to help plan for the future
• Opportunities to make decisions for himself/herself... unless safety issues begin to appear
• Discussions to have input into plans for their lives

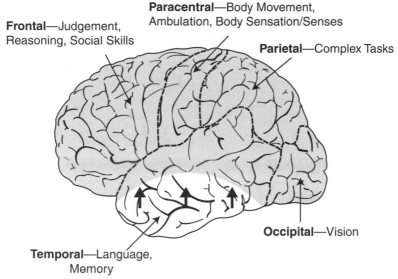

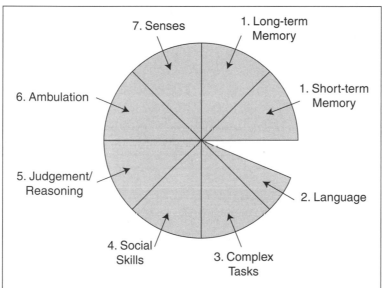

Figure 2.2   Early-to-Mild Stage. (Shaded areas show what functions remain).

- Opportunities to continue activities that give a sense of purpose to his/her life
- Situations to experience success in activities of daily living
- Comfortable spaces to share concerns and feelings with others

- Regular times to be included in family rituals and activities
- Situations to have opportunities to express his/her spirituality
- Pleasurable opportunities for stimulation of all senses
- Scheduled moments to have time to rest

Opportunities to feel accomplishment, success, and some control of his/her life are essential for the loved one's well being. There are people in the Early-to-Mild Stage who want to talk about the disease and who are willing to express their feelings and concerns. They may want to discuss their feelings about the effects the disease has on their functions and abilities. By offering them the opportunity to talk about their experiences during the diagnosis of the disease, you can learn about what he/she can still do and how they want to be treated especially in the later stages. Persons may also want to express how they see themselves as they loose some of their functions and capabilities. Examples of this are found in the book *Speaking Our Minds* by Lisa Schaefer, LCSW. She interviews persons with Alzheimer's disease and records their thoughts and feelings throughout the disease progression. Through her insight, the reader can understand the struggle of the person with the disease to communicate with words, actions, and bodily movements.

By creating environments where it is "safe" to talk about your loved one's experiences and your experiences, you are acknowledging the presence of the disease and begin to remove the stigma society places on those affected by it. To date, there have been no Alzheimer's disease survivors to talk about how the disease affected them personally and their families. Therefore, opportunities for these types of discussions need to be offered early in the disease process.

At this stage, your loved one can continue to do many things. Help him/her to realize the following and "Nurture What Remains":

1. The person can still make decisions about taking care of him/herself.
2. The person can fix meals, dress oneself, drive, carry on conversations, recognize people, do sports used to do, and so on.

3. The person can do physical activities—working and playing—if there has not been previous difficulty with hearing, seeing, and so on.
4. The person can still enjoy beauty, taking walks, going on vacations, music, and so on.
5. The person may still be able to live alone.
6. The person still needs social interaction and stimulation.
7. The person needs an environment that enables him/her to continue to function with dignity.
8. The person has the right to have others do things with him/her not necessarily for him/her.
9. The person and family members and caregivers can enjoy life together.
10. The person has the right to express his/her feelings to others and be treated as an adult and not like a child.

It can be frightening to think of the future for a person with Alzheimer's disease. Because people have the ability to self-reflect, especially in the Early Stages, the knowledge that something is not right about the way one is functioning causes worry and fear. Try to imagine the anxiety you would experience if you consistently forgot things to the point where it affected your daily life.

To the person who cannot remember the past or anticipate the future, the world around him/her can be strange and frightening.

"Unraveling the Mystery"—National Institute on Aging.

One man who was speaking to an Early Stage support group stated: "I want to have a full life. I used to be in management and had many responsibilities. I want to do meaningful work and be useful to others. Don't just give me pictures to color or cards to sort and think that I am happy. I can still do many things and do them well." Giving individuals with Alzheimer's disease an opportunity to tell their stories recognizes their worth and self-respect. It also enables society to have a deeper understanding of how the disease affects individuals and recognizes their rights of self-determination.

WHAT IS THE MODERATE STAGE? (GENERALLY A 3-TO-5 YEAR PERIOD)

Dr. Brumback discussed in depth the Moderate Stage in Chapter 1. Here are some diagrams that more fully explain the progression of Alzheimer's disease at this stage.

In the pie chart of the Moderate Stage, it is indicated that the wave of destruction has affected a greater portion of some of the functions (Figure 2.3). Long-term memory, senses, ambulation, and judgment/reasoning are unaffected, but there is little short-term memory, and there may be limited social skills, ability to do complex tasks, and language that is affected.

Moderate Stage Clues

Some of the clues that Alzheimer's disease is progressing and changes occurring are also part of the "10 Warning Signs of Alzheimer's Disease" identified in the Early-to-Mild Stage. Clues that Alzheimer's disease is progressing also take place in this stage, but they become more noticeable and frequent. The following clues have been developed by the National Alzheimer's Association.

1. Memory Changes That Disrupt Daily Life—Example: Asking for the same information repeatedly, forgetting important dates and events, and so on. Mixes up identity of people such as thinking spouse as a stranger.
2. Challenges in Planning and Solving Problems—Example: Persons may have trouble following written directions or completing tasks. The person may not be able to organize thoughts or follow logical explanations.
3. Difficulty in Completing Familiar Tasks at Home, At Work, and At Leisure—Example: The person may find it hard to complete daily tasks; trouble driving to a familiar location; managing a budget at work; or remembering the rules of a favorite game. They may have difficulty in concentrating and take much longer to do things than they did before.
4. Confusion with Time and Place—Example: Sometimes persons with Alzheimer's disease forget where they are or how they got there. They may wander and become a risk to themselves.

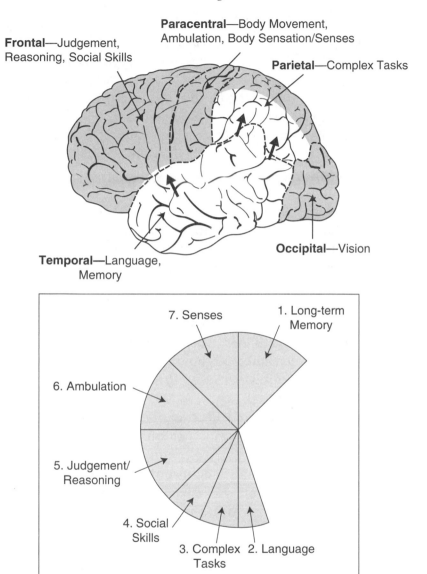

Figure 2.3   Moderate Stage. (Shaded areas show what functions remain).

5. Trouble Understanding Visual Images and Spatial Relationships—Example: They may have difficulty reading, judging distances, and determining color or contrast. In terms of perception, they may pass a mirror and think someone else is in the room. They may also have difficulty recognizing familiar objects and take things that belong to others.

6. New Problems with Words in Speaking or Writing—Example: People with Alzheimer's disease may have trouble following a conversation. They may struggle with vocabulary, have trouble finding the right word, may be able to read but cannot formulate the correct response to a written request, or call things by the wrong name.

7. Misplacing Things and Losing the Ability to Retrace Steps— Example: A person with Alzheimer's disease may put things in unusual places or may accuse others of stealing their possessions.

8. Decreased or Poor Judgment—Example: People with Alzheimer's disease may experience changes in judgment or decision making. They may use poor judgment when dealing with money, giving large amounts to telemarketers, and so on.

9. Withdrawal from Work or Social Activities—Example: People with Alzheimer's disease may start to remove themselves from hobbies, social activities, work projects, or sports. They may have trouble remembering how to work on a favorite hobby. They may withdraw because of the changes they know are occurring in themselves.

10. Changes in Mood and Personality—Example: The mood and personality of persons can quickly change. They can become confused, suspicious, depressed, fearful, or anxious and experience paranoia, delusions, or hallucinations. They may exhibit inappropriate behavior such as kicking, hitting, grabbing, and so on. Also, they may show a lack of concern for their appearance and hygiene. Sleeping may become more noticeable along with frequent naps.

In the Moderate Stage, persons with Alzheimer's disease continue to need appropriate stimulation and socialization in a safe environment. They need the following:

• Support for their sense of purpose/self-direction.... "I still can do..."
• Involvement in activities that have long been enjoyed
• Time to review one's life and celebrate what has been accomplished

- Physical exercise
- Time for rest
- A safe and predictable environment
- Stimulating all of their senses (smell, taste, touch, hearing, sight, etc.)
- Encouragement to be as productive and engaged in social activities
- Help in choosing proper clothing for the season or the occasion
- Help with handling details of toileting
- Personalized activities to stimulate and engage individuals in the Moderate Stage

You, the caregiver, need to continue to "Nurture What Remains." At this stage, the person can still do things that he/she has enjoyed throughout life.

1. The person can enjoy physical activities, if there have not been previous injuries to prohibit such activities.
2. The person can enjoy memories of the past and tell stories of his/her life.
3. The person can make decisions with assistance.
4. The person can do many tasks with "promptings" from others while gardening or heating up a meal in the microwave.
5. The person can express opinions about what he/she likes or dislikes.
6. The person can enjoy music, art, being read to, and so on.
7. The person can continue to be included in family rituals and activities.
8. The loved one should be unconditionally accepted as the person he/she is while living with dementia.
9. The person is to be allowed to have some sense of "centering," a sense of place and identity.
10. The person is to have an environment that stimulates and accommodates his/her physical and social needs.

It is important to create environments that contain clues to help persons with dementia to enhance their memory. These simple environmental changes can help persons feel competent and empowered and assist them to function independently. The environment is created by looking at the world from the perspective of the person with dementia. We must strive to change the environment to meet the needs of the person not to expect to transform the individual to suit our needs or the environment.

WHAT IS THE SEVERE STAGE?

As a caregiver, you may or may not experience this stage. Many caregivers' experiences have been that the loved one dies from cancer, stroke, heart attack, and so on and does not encounter the final stages of the disease.

This is the final stage of the disease process. At this stage, the person may lose the ability to interact properly. Persons may not be able to respond to the environment, and may have lost their ability of judgment, reasoning, and social skills. This is the stage at which many persons can no longer be managed by caregivers at home.

Survival during the Severe Stage depends a lot on the quality of nursing care, since patients lose many of the self-care functions that prevent other illnesses. Often, Alzheimer's disease is the underlying cause of death; that is, it weakens the brain control of body systems and allows other illnesses to end the person's life. Since the median survival (the time by which half the patients die) is 7 years after diagnosis, an individual may die before reaching the Severe Stage of the disease.

The pie chart representing the Severe Stage has all functions compromised except for the senses (Figure 2.4). In this advanced stage, damage to the brain's nerve cells is widespread yet there are still some areas that can be stimulated and nurtured. The pie chart indicates some of those remaining functions even though they may be very limited. Other frailties of the body will need to be taken care of as well such as hearing, sight, walking, breathing, and so on.

Severe Stage Clues

Some clues that Alzheimer's disease is progressing and changes need to occur:

1. Inability to recognize family members or faces

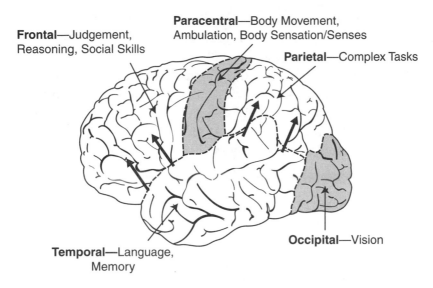

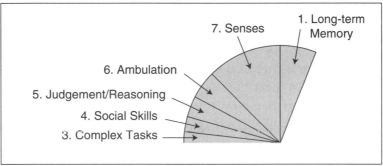

Figure 2.4   Severe Stage. (Shaded areas show what functions remain).

2. Loss of control over bodily functions and experience abnormal reflexes
3. Loss of communication although words or phrases may occasionally be uttered
4. Loss of capacity to respond to their environment
5. May experience increased vulnerability to other diseases
6. May refuse to eat, chokes, or forgets to swallow
7. Needs total assistance for all activities of daily living

At this stage, caregivers need to be true "detectives." They must "read" body language as well as listen attentively to any words that are expressed to understand and accommodate their loved one's wishes and needs. This stage can be the most difficult for family members and caregivers as they begin to focus on the comfort of their loved ones rather than on prolonging their life. They begin to address end-of-life issues talking about and working through their grief. This can also be a time when the caregiver experiences feelings of guilt and feelings of failure. The feeling is often like "We have cared for our loved one for so long and done everything we knew how and still our loved one is suffering."

Persons with Alzheimer's disease continue to need the presence of others (socialization), some stimulation of the senses, and a safe environment. They also need:

- To have their wishes, preferences, and decisions respected by others
- To be cared for by individuals well-trained in dementia care
- To be kept free from pain
- To receive stimulation of the senses—sight, taste, smell, and especially touch (hands, feet, hugs, and kisses, if accepted)
- To have visits of a spiritual leader if the person wants it
- To be in a safe and predictable, loving environment that is tailored to meet their special needs
- To be cherished for all that the person is
- To be given understanding and compassion so that a person has a sense of leaving this world ... even though he/she may not speak of it

The progression of Alzheimer's disease across the brain has affected almost all bodily systems. Most of the 10 Warning Signs are present. Yet, the person can still enjoy the following:

1. The person can still enjoy stories of the past.
2. The person can make known his/her opinions about eating, drinking, music, and conversation.
3. The person can still enjoy being touched if it was acceptable in the past.
4. The person can enjoy company—about one or two people at a time. The person may or may not recognize others by name but will feel the visitors' presence.
5. The person can continue to enjoy prayers, poems, music, and so on.

6. The person should be reminded about the good he/she has done in life.
7. The person can enjoy the presences of others.
8. The person can enjoy nature or just sitting by a sunny window.
9. The caregivers can read newspapers, books, hymns, and prayers.
10. The caregivers can play favorite movies or have favorite music playing during quiet times.
11. The "enduring self" is still present and should be nourished.

As verbal communication decreases, through careful observation, it is essential to be aware of behaviors or to piece together parts of speech in order to connect with the person. Every person diagnosed with Alzheimer's disease or a dementia has individual rights. Reflecting on these rights can help caregivers adjust their caregiving to recognize the person's dignity throughout the progression of the disease and to "Nurture What Remains."

When one puts together all the information on the stages, one knows that our society has much to learn about how to care for persons with Alzheimer's disease and other dementia. People with Alzheimer's disease may not move through all stages. They may have contributing physical ailments and complications that may alter the course of the disease. However, staging of the illness gives us guidelines for assessment and helping us understand the progression of the disease. We have collapsed the disease progression into three stages in order to make it easier to conceptualize the disease process and to plan for continuous care that would maximize the person's functions throughout life.

CHAPTER 3

The Enduring Self

Connie Kudlacek

As a caregiver, you will find this statement to be true: "If you have met one person with Alzheimer's disease, you have met *one* person with Alzheimer's disease." That sentence expresses the "mystery" of working with and relating with the personal world of every individual person, but especially when relating with persons who have some type of dementia. This statement exemplifies the reality that the disease process affects each person in a distinctive way, making it difficult to develop "step-by-step" procedures for their care. Although there are commonalities, individuals with Alzheimer's disease experience the disease uniquely. The deterioration does not occur in a lockstep manner.

Persons with dementia have varying abilities to communicate with the world outside them because of how their individual brain is affected by the disease. They communicate differently as the disease progresses— sometimes with words; sometimes with "babble"; and sometimes with gestures, art, dance, smiles, frowns, and vacant eyes. An example of babbling was given in the introduction where the women babbled but sang hymns in church perfectly.

Generally, persons with dementia respond to and remember LOVE. Love can be expressed in many ways, but the challenge is to continue to love a person who is changing because of a disease process. Little children usually give unconditional love. Can we move to that place within our lives where we as caregivers can mimic a child's unconditional love for others?

Dr. Sam Fazio has written a book titled *The Enduring Self in People with Alzheimer's: Getting to the Heart of Individualized Care*. He states that even though some skills are lost, the enduring self of the person is present. The "enduring self" means the ongoing or lifelong person and this concept is perfect when thinking of a person with dementia. The person or self is always there even though many of his/her functions may be compromised by the disease process. Persons with Alzheimer's disease need to be treated with dignity and respect at all times. They also are wondering what is happening in their lives, especially as they experience the early stages of Alzheimer's disease.

Try putting yourself in the place of the person with Alzheimer's disease:

- Try to imagine the anxiety when a person thinks, "I don't know why I said that."
- Try to imagine what it must be like when a person begins consistently to get lost while driving and can't find his or her way home.
- Try to imagine what it is like to be aware that you can no longer take care of paying bills and other financial matters.
- Try to imagine what it is like to make plans to go out to a show or to dinner, but then consistently forget to show up.
- Try to imagine being in a room full of people who know you but you do not have a clue as to who some of them are.

Following is a chart of the Preserved Functions and Abilities of the person with dementia as the disease progresses across the brain (Figure 3.1). This chart, prepared by Dr. Roger A. Brumback and revised in 2010, shows the progression of the disease and the functions or capabilities that remain in each stage of the disease.

As you review the chart keep in mind that even though some functions become weak and even lost, the person still remains with some functions and abilities and enjoyment of the senses and wants to be in control of his/her life. This is the "enduring self." The implications of this chart are that by understanding the remaining functions you can maximize the person's abilities and preserve his/her dignity by offering supportive treatments. Being aware of what functions may remain allows you a new perspective on opportunities to implement ways to bring dignity and supportive treatments to your loved one's life. All involved in this process must be flexible and open to change.

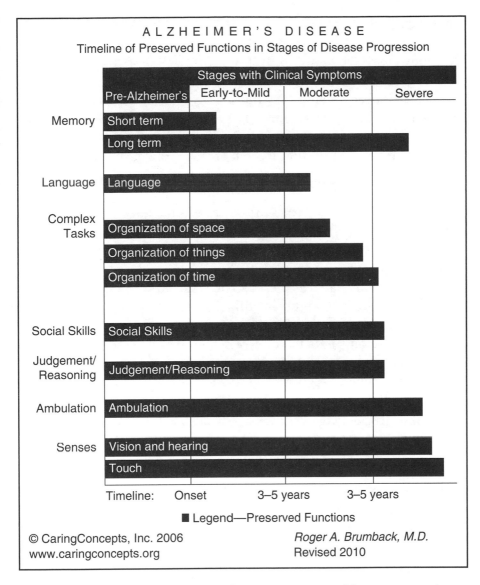

Figure 3.1   Timeline of preserved functions in stages of disease progression.

What is "supportive treatment" for Alzheimer's disease? In the book *Alzheimer's Disease—The Dignity Within: A Handbook for Caregivers, Family, and Friends,* Dr. Brumback gives an answer to this question: "Education of the affected individual, caregivers, family, and friends regarding both the lost and the preserved brain functions is part of a 'supportive therapy program'. Instead of focusing on deficits, the focus should be on the preserved abilities and the development of compensatory strategies." Caregivers need to look at the glass as being half full rather than half empty. Hope is a powerful drug—not only for those living with Alzheimer's disease but also for those who care for them.

Dr. Brumback stated that the best treatment for persons with Alzheimer's disease is to support the functions that remain in the brain ... as if someone were helping boost the brain's functions as with the use of a "spare tire" to help an automobile continue to move along. This image tells us that what remains can be supported and enhanced with "individual" proper care. Those caring for the person with dementia need to strive for "unconditional acceptance" of the person as to where he/she is in the disease process.

The word *power* in its Greek form means "ability" and "capacity." When the word power is used in this book, it refers to the knowledge individuals have, as well as their capacity to choose wisely. This type of education process will then give the caregiver the tools and choices to "Nurture What Remains."

Every person wants to be in control of his or her life. It is confusing to the person with Alzheimer's disease and to family members who become caregivers to see someone function normally on many things and then to not be able to do some of the things one used to do. Often persons find ways to cover-up and compensate for functions that are becoming weak. The symptoms of Alzheimer's disease are not just lapses in memory but a combination of criteria that hinder the person's daily activities. No single behavior can be called characteristic or diagnostic of Alzheimer's disease. However, an individual who has several behavioral symptoms likely is experiencing something other than just the normal brain aging process.

These changes usually are not sudden, but slowly and progressively become more apparent over many months... years. While it is not likely that caregivers and persons with dementia will be able to look inside a living brain, we have to base our judgments on signs, symptoms, and behaviors of people with Alzheimer's disease to determine what stage of the disease process they are in. While the symptoms have been classified into stages, there is no way to determine how long each stage will last.

By using the staging process, we are able to distinguish a time span in the disease process and then begin to recognize abilities that remain rather than losses that have taken place. Staging helps us facilitate transitions in a compassionate way by giving us clues to find ways for the person to have control over his/her life. Caregivers and family members can maximize the person's abilities and preserve his or her dignity, which in turn allows him/her to "succeed." Staging is not being specific. It is not clearly a black and white process but always a gray area where the caregiver must observe behaviors. Staging of the illness can serve the purpose of providing "clues" and "cues" for making plans for continuous care.

Current research is being done today to find a cure for the disease. But until a cure is found, families, caregivers, and friends of persons with dementia are the only ones who can support each individual in his/her particular progression with the disease. The needs of the caregiver evolve over time; therefore, information about the disease needs to be geared to the different stages of the disease and more research needs to be done in the area of supportive treatments.

The Resources for Enhancing Alzheimer's Caregiver Health (REACH) has published the results of a clinical trial, which showed that caregivers who received 6 months of intensive help with caregiving strategies had significant improvements in overall quality of life. These caregivers reported that taking part in the REACH program helped them feel more confident in working with their loved one, made life easier for them, improved their caregiving ability, improved the care recipient's life, and helped them keep their loved one at home. These caregivers also had lower rates of clinical depression compared with caregivers who did not participate in the program (*Alzheimer's Disease: Unraveling the Mystery from the National Institute on Aging*).

Research along with reports by caregivers on their experiences has shown that there can be positive outcomes of caregiving. Some of those are:

- Opportunity to build a stronger relationship with a spouse or loved one
- Opportunity to repay a person for previous actions
- Opportunity to strengthen family ties
- Opportunity to reintroduce family rituals and activities

- Opportunity to reach out to others and develop a broad base of support
- Opportunity to renew religious/spiritual conviction

When we put together all of this information, we know that our society has much to learn about how to care for persons with Alzheimer's disease and other dementia. We believe some of the most important things we can do to help those caregivers, family, and friends of persons with dementia are the following:

- Develop ways to help them become knowledgeable about Alzheimer's disease.
- Show the effect of the progression of the disease on the person's abilities and functions. (This is like putting together the pieces of the complex puzzle of Alzheimer's disease.)
- Help them make appropriate choices.
- Alert caregivers to finding "cues" and "clues" when transitions for caregiving occur.
- Help caregivers take care of themselves in the process of looking after their loved ones.
- Help caregivers to experience acceptance of what is happening in the present moment.
- "Nurture What Remains" in those with Alzheimer's disease.

So let us present to you a simple analogy that was given by Timothy R. Malloy, MD, Associate Professor/Director of Geriatrics, Department of Family Medicine at the University of Nebraska Medical Center. Dr. Malloy is known for his ability to simplify a person's care through a common sense approach to his or her medical, as well as his or her personal, care. This analogy is not meant to be disrespectful or trivialize the ordeal of Alzheimer's disease, but only to be used as an educational base to show how the predictability of Alzheimer's disease plays out. Dr. Malloy states, "In order to wage a fight, it's helpful to know that you are in a fight and what the rules are."

Like a football game, we can segregate the progression of Alzheimer's disease into four quarters. But a football game has four equal quarters, and we know that no one person who has Alzheimer's disease is affected the same, so let's go with some general rules of play (Figure 3.2).

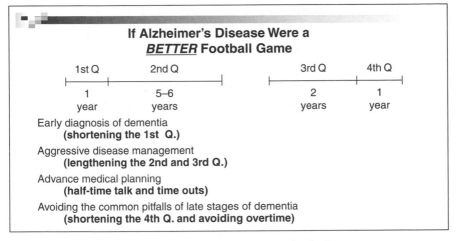

Figure 3.2   If Alzheimer's disease were a better football game.

As a caregiver, the overall goals when using this analogy are:

- To have the healthcare professional see the person with Alzheimer's disease early in the disease process
- To lengthening out the 2nd and 3rd quarters through aggressive disease management
- To slow the rate of deterioration, therefore increasing the time of cognition and functioning
- To adequately have time for advanced planning
- To adequately communicate during the half-time talks about prognostic information with a likely time frame
- To limit the duration and suffering of the 4th quarter
- To make an impact on how the disease plays out
- To plan, communicate, and initiate hospice to help limit the painful 4th quarter
- To apply the serenity prayer

God grant me the serenity to accept the things I cannot change; courage to change the things I can; and wisdom to know the difference.

—Reinhold Niebuhr

By coming to grips with the problems early and seeking out a diagnosis, the individuals with Alzheimer's disease and their families can initiate treatments along with other coexisting conditions. According to the Alzheimer's Association, some of the benefits of an early diagnosis of Alzheimer's disease are:

- Current care concepts and medical treatments can help maintain the person's level of independence longer.
- The person with dementia has the ability to participate in the planning for his/her future and care options.
- There is time to develop relationships with medical professionals and the "care team."
- The person may choose to participate in clinical drug trials.
- There is time to benefit from care options making it easier for the person and family to manage the disease process.

By tapping into the benefits of an early diagnosis, the person with dementia and the caregiver can then prepare to lengthen the 2nd and 3rd quarters by treating the disease. These quarters or time periods are similar to the Early-to-Mild and Moderate Stages of the disease where the person with Alzheimer's disease still has retained much of his/her functional ability, especially in the Early-to-Mild Stage. Again it is in those two quarters where the greatest opportunity to "Nurture What Remains" exists. You may want to review Figure 3.1 that outlines the preserved functions in the stages of disease progression in order to better understand this concept.

Finally in the 4th quarter caregivers, at this stage, often fail to recognize the other contributing health issues that are coming into play such as weight loss and pneumonia resulting in initiating aggressive medical treatments. The question that needs to be asked at this time is, "What would your loved one want you to do if he or she could advise you now?" Using the Football Game analogy, families should have had a discussion about the end-of-life issues in the first two quarters of the game or when the person first begins to have some functional decline. In these open discussions, a Healthcare Power of Attorney can be identified who will make decisions that are consistent with the individual's expressed wishes for care. But experience has shown that these discussions often do not take place, and if they do they often only touch on Cardiac Pulmonary Resuscitation status. Absence of open communication about end-of-life issues leaves everyone in a dilemma. Dr. Malloy says that planning, prognostic communications, and the initiation of the idea of hospice can help to limit the painful 4th quarter.

Hospice is a choice that can allow the 4th quarter to come to an end as painlessly as possible for all. In hospice care, aggressive life-sustaining treatments are normally not recommended. Aggressive life sustaining treatments such as artificial nutrition and hydrations, cardiopulmonary resuscitation or antibiotics may seem cruel to individuals with dementia because of their lack of ability to understand the use of these treatment and their lack of orientation to the moment.

Additionally, we know that success at football is only gained when using a "team approach" with strong leadership or a team captain. This perspective of a team is also useful when dealing with the responsibilities of caring for a loved one who has Alzheimer's disease and other dementia.

Persons with dementia also can find comfort knowing that a team of individuals can understand their special needs and care for them when the primary caregiver may not be available. The team of caregivers can also offer opportunities for stimulation and socialization, encouraging persons to use their remaining functions in different ways. An example of this stimulation was a situation where a respite care volunteer, Henry, came to my father-in-law's home weekly to visit, play some music, and talk about steam engines. Henry was close to my father-in-law's age and had farmed with steam engines so they both had a lot to talk about. Even when my father-in-law was not able to easily communicate, he always seemed to get excited when Henry came to visit. Later in the disease process, my father-in-law was very comfortable allowing his wife to leave for appointments as long as Henry was there with him.

In this situation, "person-centered" care was the focus. Even though the primary caregiver was able to take a day off to re-energize herself, my father-in-law was treated as an individual with interests and memories, provided a positive social environment, and recognized for things he had accomplished in life. Henry, the volunteer, connected with his client and continued to stimulate the enduring self within.

CHAPTER 4

Watch Out! Potential Financial Exploitation or Abuse

Juli-Ann Gasper

Financial exploitation/abuse of older adults is becoming more prevalent in our society. For older adults who are more vulnerable because of Alzheimer's disease or related dementia, financial exploitation/abuse by someone else is very easy. We point out this possible danger for your loved one so that you as a caregiver can protect your loved one from such abuse.

POTENTIAL DANGERS

Every reader of this book now knows what it feels like to not understand where your money went and how to get along in the future. After the financial crisis of 2009, we are all more cognizant of the importance of managing the financial resources we have. For an elderly person or vulnerable adult who can't go back into the work force to replace lost money, loss of funds is life-changing. When the funds were lost due to financial exploitation, the sense of betrayal and inability to understand how one could have been so vulnerable make these losses particularly heartbreaking.

An elder whose funds have been taken without permission may be left without resources for needed medical care and food, inability to do maintenance and repairs on the home (often the person's biggest asset), and a mistrust of all those who come and go in his/her life. As a caregiver, you have intimate contact with the elder. You may know that you did not abscond with funds or misuse resources, but an elder with dementia does not know that.

Many studies of elder abuse suggest that financial exploitation is the predominant form of abuse. The stories that make it to the media are stunning; more than 60 percent of elder abuse reports are financial. In just the first 6 months of 2009, newspapers around the US reported over $50 million of elder financial exploitation, not including the highly publicized cases of Bernard Madoff (exploiter) and Brooke Astor (exploited). The average loss in financial abuses that made it to the papers was almost $275,000. There is no accurate estimate of the number of victims or the losses because they are not big enough to make it to the newspaper. Police departments tell us that financial exploitation is the largest category of complaints filed by elders or their legal representatives.

Who are the exploiters? The majority are not strangers. More than 70 percent are known to the elder: 23 percent are relatives, 18 percent are in-home caregivers, 6 percent are friends and neighbors, 16 percent are professional advisors and service providers, and 14 percent are institutional employees.

You probably already understand some of the frustrations and complications of managing someone else's financial resources. How easy it could be to step over the line. This chapter aims to help you understand the financial capabilities of persons with Alzheimer's disease so as to optimize the use of financial resources to make life the best it can be for both you and the person for whom you care.

What reasons do exploiters cite for using funds in less than honest ways? A very common argument is this: "I am the beneficiary of the estate anyway. I need the money now. Why should I have to wait?" If I am happier, she will be happier, too. Another argument is the entitlement claim: "I am doing all this work for him and not getting compensated. It is just reasonable to think that I should be able to fill my gas tank and buy my groceries on his dime. Lack of participation by other family members is often cited as justification for taking over management of funds." They just refuse to get involved and I'm the one doing all the work. This at least makes me feel like I am not being exploited myself! Often dysfunctionality in families leads to financially exploitive behavior against the elder.

We want to help you recognize what financial capacities your loved one has and make use of those capabilities to optimize the lives of both you and your loved one. We offer insights to help you better understand your role as a financial caregiver during different phases of the disease. We will try to help you design safeguards for yourself, your family member with dementia, and other family members and neighbors to prevent financial exploitation.

HOW ALZHEIMER'S DISEASE CHANGES FINANCIAL CAPABILITIES

Impairments in financial skills and judgment are often the first functional changes demonstrated by persons who have Alzheimer's disease or other dementia. The changes occur irregularly, often quickly, out of the sequence you expected—perhaps unpredictably. There are several steps. First, you may realize that she can make decisions about this particular financial situation, but can't really do it herself. Later, she may delegate the task to you and say, "You just go ahead and do it for me, Jennie." Eventually you'll find that she really isn't aware that it needs to be done. The speed of regression differs from person to person and task to task.

AWARENESS BY PERSONS WITH ALZHEIMER'S DISEASE OF FINANCIAL LOSSES TAKING PLACE

Your loved one has differing levels of awareness of what is going on in her brain. She probably knows that she is not in complete control of what is going on. The self-knowledge that she is forgetting things or does not always understand makes her more vulnerable to suggestions that are not in her best interest. She may be overly excited at the chance to make a decision for herself once again—even if it is the wrong decision.

Your loved one has most likely lost the ability to anticipate consequences. As his brain changes, your father may be able to understand the specific transaction being suggested, but not the consequences of that action as they relate to other aspects of his financial affairs.

- For example, a charity asks for a donation. He understands what they say and what they are going to do with the money and thinks it is a good cause. He knows where the checkbook is and how to write a check, so he donates $5,000, even though there isn't that much in his account. When the check bounces, a legitimate charity would call back and try to figure out how to make things right. An exploiter would just cash the check and disappear, leaving your father to deal with the bank, the overdraft penalties, his own confusion about what happened, and his shame at having been duped.

- For example, your father knows he can no longer negotiate a trip to get cash from the bank and that someone else will have to do that for him. He may not know how to decide who is trustworthy to do that for him or the best way to make it happen without exploitation. His neighbor conveniently offers to do it. He starts to write a check for the neighbor to take to the bank for cash and the neighbor says, "Oh, you know, it would be a lot easier and faster if I just took your ATM card. Then I won't have to park and go into the bank and all that hassle." Your father is most grateful for the offer and doesn't want to cause any trouble and agrees that it would indeed be easier that way. The neighbor now has access to both the card and the PIN number.

A third aspect concerns the willingness of persons with Alzheimer's disease to communicate their own awareness that understanding of financial affairs has decreased. All our lives, we use "little white lies" to explain something when we don't want to reveal the "real reason." This is learned social behavior from a very early age.

- For example, Mary's father asked her to help him balance the checkbook every month, citing his macular degeneration as the reason. But perhaps it was really that he realized he couldn't do that task anymore; after all, he could still see well enough to pay the bills and open the mail. Balancing the checkbook is a task that requires different mental skills than paying bills and reading the mail.

The second issue here is that if you are able to discern what the underlying reason is that he is turning over the task to someone else, it may help explain some other things going on. In this example, any task that requires comparing amounts between two sources might be a source of frustration. Your awareness helps you to be supportive of activities that are straightforward, while moving out of his sphere of influence those activities that he can no longer do.

NURTURE WHAT REMAINS: FINANCIAL MANAGEMENT SKILLS AND KNOWLEDGE

The research literature about changes in financial management skills during the different stages of Alzheimer's disease is sparse and new. Very little has been "measured" or "quantified" to help us understand what skills remain the longest and which ones typically disappear earlier. What follows is my own interpretation of the results from three research groups who have studied this question in the last 10 years.

Let us examine some of the items in Figure 4.1.

Set 1: Basic Monetary Skills include being able to manipulate coins and currency: identification, counting, and relative values and being able to put

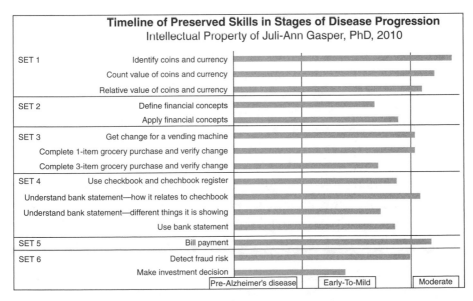

Figure 4.1 Financial Management Perspective.

together a certain sum. At least two of these (identification and counting) are probably "overlearned" skills that go way back to early childhood and as such, remain quite a long time into the disease. So taking advantage of these capabilities might include such things as:

- "Mom, could you get my billfold and pull out $5 so we can pay for the _____ when it gets delivered this morning?"
- Each day your father goes through the coins received in change yesterday and separates out the quarters because that is what is needed for the washing machines in the apartment building.
- Together you make a decision that all the dimes this year will be set aside and used as gifts for the seven grandchildren at the holidays. You make an envelope with each grandchild's name on it. When you have separated out seven dimes, one goes in each envelope. You talk about each grandchild as you are putting the dime in his or her envelope. You talk about what your loved one used dimes for when she was a child. What could a dime buy in those days? Talk about the depression: "Brother, can you spare a dime?" You record these stories and they are given to the grandchildren along with the dimes.

Set 2: This set is defining and applying Financial Concepts. It may seem odd that the ability to apply financial concepts probably lasts longer than being able to define them. The idea here is that he knows he gets interest on his savings account, but gradually loses the ability to explain why and how the interest calculation works. He just knows he gets the interest.

Set 3: The third set relates to Cash Transactions.

- "Hi, Mary. This is Mom. I want to get a soda from the machine but I don't have any coins. Can you bring me some?" "Well, good morning, Mom. Did you sleep well last night? . . . Have you talked to your neighbor Helen this morning? . . . Maybe she has some coins that she can trade you for a dollar bill."

The research shows that there is a definite difference in the ability to carry out a one-item purchase and the ability to do a similar transaction with three items. This could be helpful for you to know when giving your loved one a list of things to do or buy. If you have perceived that she is able to do a three-item list without confusion, then always give three things to do. If you find that she can really only keep one item at a time in her mind, you'll both be much less frustrated if you respect that limitation and build your interactions around that knowledge.

- Perhaps you organize the grocery list into small "post it" notes with three items from one aisle grouped together on one note. She doesn't have to wander around the store getting distracted and can enjoy the sense of accomplishment as you together crumple up the note and say "There! That's done! Thanks, Mom!" Then give her another set to find. "Here, Mom, would you like to look for our breakfast cereals?"

Set 4: Using a Checkbook, Checkbook Register, and Bank Statements is the fourth group of skills in the figure. The general concepts of "checkbook register" and "bank statement" may be familiar longer than the ability to actually manipulate the information.

- "Did you get your bank statement in the mail, yesterday, Mom?" is a different question "level" than "How much money do you have in the bank?" which is different from "When was your last deposit?"
- Identifying information on the bank statement or finding specific transactions probably is a skill that is preserved longer than being able to reconcile the bank statement and the checkbook. Again, comparison between two documents is harder to do than working with just one document.
- A lot of bank statement and checkbook activities involve arithmetic processes. Being able to do arithmetic is one of those skills that are lost by people at vastly different rates and timeframes. Your loved one may be unable to add a column of numbers but can still add two numbers. So you structure the task as sets of two numbers rather than presenting a whole column that may seem overwhelming and impossible.

Set 5: Bill Paying is a task none of us likes to do and it is often complicated, complex, and tedious. At the end of this chapter,

I have experimented with a checklist approach. My list of the steps involved in bill paying quickly approaches 20! Each task has a different combination of mobility requirements, memory and spatial understanding, fine motor skills, concept understanding, and use of the senses. And yet, many of the skills needed are preserved in the Early-to-Mild Stage. As a caregiver, you'll want to help her retain these skills as long as possible.

Set 6: Detection of Fraud Risk skills include being able to recognize when someone else has been scammed or defrauded, being able to identify and talk about signs of fraud, and being able to recognize those signs in her own situation. Every time you can bring up an example of someone being defrauded and have a discussion (two-way, not one-way!), this will help to preserve the fraud risk detection capabilities a little longer.

- Discuss news reports of financial exploitations. It is not necessary for this to be "preachy." Don't "should" on her. The discussion can have lots of back-and-forth comments between you and your loved one. "Did you hear about the guy in Kansas who . . . ? What was he thinking? Have you heard of this happening around here? How did the scammer make the scheme work?" Allow your parent to educate you! "Mom, why would he do that?" This will allow you to perceive your loved one's conceptual, pragmatic, and judgmental capabilities, and over time, to recognize changes.

Another aspect of fraud detection involves the recognition of the importance of asking for advice if she isn't sure whether something is a good idea. You can help to create an environment in which questioning and talking through decisions is considered to be okay and important.

- If you ask her opinion on financial decisions you are making, it establishes a routine of the two of you talking about financial things before acting. Starting these discussions very early in the disease process will make it easier for you to see when understanding financial concepts decrease.

- ▪ "Mom, John and I met with the bank today to see if we should _____. Did you and Dad ever do that? … How did it work out? …"
- • You might put up a note by the telephone with a script for her to use when someone calls about a contribution or purchase. "Remember yesterday when that guy from _____ called to see if you wanted to buy a _____? You were kind of annoyed because you didn't really know what to say. So I made this note for you to use when someone calls and asks you to buy something or give them some money. Just read the note to the caller so he will know that you want to talk to me before you decide what to do. I'll put it right here on the wall by the telephone."

Set 7: Making Investment Decisions is probably among the most stressful of financial activities. Again, there are numerous dimensions to this domain of decision making. In most cases, you won't actually be doing many calculations, so your father's ability to talk about investments may last much longer than you might have guessed. However, decisions about lump sums or monthly income withdrawals may be much more difficult to comprehend. If your family situation is peaceful and cordial and cooperative, the discussion will be much easier. If there is dysfunctionality, it may make sense for you to "assign" this realm of decisions to one person and just avoid the discussions! Nothing gets people more heated up than talking about money!

WHAT ARE THE BEST WAYS TO WORK WITH YOUR LOVED ONE REGARDING FINANCES?

You have to decide from the beginning (and make many new decisions along the way) what you can do and what you cannot do. As a caregiver, it is not likely that you can do everything! Accept that truth and determine the best way to allow yourself to be of the best service to your loved one.

- • I have a PhD in finance and taught Personal Financial Management for many years. However, I delegated my dad's financial record-keeping and bill paying to one of my cousins. Why? Dad needed my physical presence and social support. I chose to focus my caregiving on those two things. It doesn't take a PhD to pay the bills and balance the bank statement. We paid my cousin to do the work, and I was able to reduce the number of hours per week that I needed to be involved with Dad. I was much less resentful of all the work when I could focus my energies on just being there.

• An additional aspect of this decision was that Dad was always apologetic that he was "causing so much trouble." Removing this one source of "trouble" from his mind was very freeing for him. Any time he mentioned it, I'd say, "It's no trouble, Dad. Nancy is doing it!" We'd get a little chuckle out of that and go on to the next topic. He never made the connection that he was sorry for causing trouble for Nancy!

• Before I made this arrangement with Nancy, I would be sitting with Dad wishing I were at home doing the finances, because I knew it would take me several hours. When at home doing the finances, I would be thinking I should be home with Dad.

You might ask why I didn't just do all the financial stuff while I was at Dad's place. Good question! Dad was in assisted living and later a nursing facility, with staff and visitors in and out of his apartment all the time. He and I, together, made the decision that it was safer for him to not have a check book and credit card and cash sitting around in plain sight. It gave us an opportunity to discuss theft of money or credit cards, identity theft, and misuse of funds. He was quite happy to not have to worry about those things any longer. He knew there was an issue, but not how to deal with it.

In the Early-to-Mild Stage of Alzheimer's disease, it is best to help the person with Alzheimer's to retain control of his life and for you to act as a resource person to assist him as needed.

In this phase, there may be little need for you to systematically evaluate what skills he has and what tasks he is capable of doing. It may be enough to simply ask periodically, "Is there anything you want me to help with in your money matters?" He is still in charge; it is up to him to tell you when help is necessary. Probably your biggest task in this stage is to be observant so that you pay attention to losses in capabilities or understanding and warning signs of exploitation, such as:

- Cash withdrawals that don't seem to be warranted or needed
- Checks being written at a time of the month when bill paying is not going on; that is, out of normal routine
- She is talking about making home repairs or maintenance that are not really necessary
- She is becoming really close to a young person who has no logical connection to the family
- Frequent visits from (or to) a financial advisor or lender when there really is no business that needs to be conducted
- Long phone calls where he is just basically listening and not really taking part in a two-way conversation, especially if there is a follow-up call or visit scheduled

A second function you can serve is that of "discussion leader." Think about how we keep knowledge, information, and opinions fresh and interesting. If you never discuss politics, then your knowledge of the "players" and the issues will decline. However, every time you participate in a political discussion, you bring to the forefront of your mind the knowledge, information, and opinions that you have created in the past. The same will be true for financial management. If the last time you and your loved one talked about identity theft was when you were a teenager with your first credit card and your parent (the one you are now a caregiver for) lectured you about never letting someone else use your credit card, then that topic is deeply buried. To bring it back to the top of the pile, you need to talk about it. Start the conversation.

The caregiving style that assists the loved one to be in control for as long as possible probably dominates during the earliest stages of the disease. This is also the time when your loved one is more capable of telling you what he or she wants out of life. Take advantage of that time to discuss and organize things.

Ask if she needs help organizing her documents and then follow through if she says "yes." The documents could include estate plans, wills, power of attorney agreements, investment statements, insurance policies, bank statements, birth certificates, marriage license, passport, armed service papers, funeral arrangements, receipts for paid funeral and cemetery plots, and so on. Help her maintain her routine. If she has always paid the bills on the 1st of the month, make it a ritual to continue her practice. If you know that she likes to go to the bank on Mondays, help keep track of Mondays and remind her during your Sunday afternoon visit that tomorrow is Monday and talk about the bank trip and what she will do when she is there. Help her make a list and tuck it in her wallet.

MODERATE STAGE

When you move into the Moderate Stage, you may be doing a lot more of the decision making if you are the Power of Attorney for Finances. You bring your own personal characteristics, your own preferred style of money management, your own knowledge, organizational practices, and skills into the situation. Because you are becoming more intimately involved in the details, you will naturally want to structure some of the activities in ways that are most comfortable for you, but this may not match the way your loved one has always done it. In this stage, the person can still explain how she likes things done. She can still do many of the actual tasks, with your guidance.

In some cases, you may decide to take on the role of the "assistant."

- For example, to help your mother pay the bills, you might go through them ahead of time and use a highlighter in her favorite color to locate the due date, the amount owed, and the payee. Then, when she sits down to pay the bill, she will be able to find that information "on her own."
- You might offer to actually write out the checks for him as he tells you the payee, date, and amount, leaving him to sign them. The signing of checks has a symbolic meaning to most of us; that we are in charge: "Well, he's the one who signs the checks, so I guess he is in charge here!"
- You may ask Mom to tell you what things need to be done and make a list. She is the one making the list. You are just recording it on paper. Discussion of the items can occur while this is

happening. "I need to talk to the lawyer." "Okay, I'll put that on the list. What should I tell him is the purpose of the appointment? ... Oh, really? Why did you decide to do that?"

In some cases, you use your questions to prompt Mother about things that need to get done and who will do them and to make sure that you have information YOU need to be supportive in decision making.

- "Mom, you said yesterday that you wanted to pay bills today. Should I get everything ready for that?"
- "Hey, Dad, the calendar says there is a meeting today at the Senior Center. Do you still want to go? Do you know who is talking and what the topic is? ... Oh, really? I didn't realize you were considering taking out a reverse mortgage on the house. Maybe I should go too so I can learn about it." If you go too, then it will be easier to say, later on, "No, I think what he meant by that was that if you ... then..." Or "I'm thinking we ought to get another opinion on that question. What he said didn't make sense to me." This last interaction allows your loved one to agree that he does not really understand it either, without it being seen as admitting defeat to the disease. Remind him that the wisest among us are often those who know what they DON'T know.

Don't become an enabler by taking over tasks that your loved one can still do.

- If she can still understand her bank statement, then just monitor what is going on, rather than "looking over her shoulder" as she is working with it.
- If she can still count out the grocery money, she should keep that task. Referring to the Preserved Skills chart for Financial Management, you can see that the tasks relating to coins and currency are preserved much longer into the disease than is investment decision making.

It is interesting to note that conceptual understanding continues far longer than actual decision-making ability.

- He still follows the stock market news on television and can intelligently (as much as any of us) discuss the economy, but does not understand how to make decisions about his investments.

When you are working together, talk about what you are doing and why or how. Ask questions. Help him feel that he is an active participant in the activity and decision making. Have your loved one do his/her part and you do your part.

- Balancing the checkbook: your loved one may be able to read the check to you while you find it in the statement or record the transaction.
- Bill paying:
  - She finds all the information and you write it on the check because her fine motor skills aren't so good anymore.
  - She writes out the check for bill paying while you find and tell her the amount, the vendor name, and the date. In other words, she fills in the blanks while you find the data needed.

As you continue to assist your loved one, you are "Nurturing What Remains" in the area of finances for your loved one. Because each person's brain changes in different ways, we can't say that one particular skill goes before the other. As you begin to notice changes, it might be very useful to think about the multiple steps involved in financial management task.

For example, a person does not, all of a sudden, lose the ability to write a check. There are at least four or five processes: locating the checkbook; figuring out the data that goes on the check (date, payee, amount in dollars, amount in words, and signature); locating the right place to put each piece of data; being able to actually do the handwriting on the check; and verifying the information. These steps tap into different sections of the brain and it is quite likely that they disappear from the repertoire in different sequence and time frame for different people.

Paying bills is a complex multistep process. Think about which steps your loved one can still do! Help your loved one in the bill paying process as long as you can. "Nurture What Remains" in order to give him/her dignity in accomplishing the task. Here is a list of 15 steps needed to complete the task of paying a bill. You'll probably be able to think of several more steps that I have forgotten. Can your loved one still do the following?

1. Retrieve the mail from the mailbox. (Is mobile enough to do this; doesn't get lost on the way to or from; understands how to open the mailbox.)

2. Open an envelope. (Can figure out which place on the envelope to pull to get it open; has the fine motor skill dexterity to open it without ripping the contents; doesn't sustain multiple, hard-to-heal, paper cuts.)

3. Separate the bill and the return envelope from the advertising inserts. (Can visually distinguish between the ads and the bill itself; understands how to make two piles.)

4. Trash the advertising inserts. (Knows where the trash can or paper recycling bin is; is mobile enough to do this task.)

5. Locate the important parts of the bill. (Date due, amount, address, etc.) (Still has good reading skills and eyesight.)

6. Retrieve the checkbook from its "home." (Remembers where it is kept and how to get there; is mobile enough to do this.)

7. Fill out the check with appropriate information.

8. Pair the check and the bill stub to put into the envelope, making sure the address shows through the front address window. (Understands the construction of an envelope and how to place the address portion so it shows; understands that the check has to go behind the bill stub; understands how to turn the envelope over to see if the address shows through.)

9. Lick the envelope and close it AFTER inserting the bill stub and the check. (Can stick her tongue out and can lick the right place! Understands the "AFTER" sequence.)

10. Retrieve the postage stamps from their "home." (Remembers where they are stored and is mobile enough to get there.)

11. Figure out amount of postage needed. (Remembers the first class postage rate.)

12. Figure out which stamps to use to get that amount of postage. (Understands relative value of stamps and can add them up to get the right amount.)

13. Can lick the stamps or remove them from the backing sheet (Can stick her tongue out. Has fine motor skills needed to remove a stamp from a backing sheet.)
14. Knows where to put the stamps on the envelope.
15. Take the envelope to the mailbox.

Obviously, your loved ones ability to complete the tasks on this list will change over time, so make sure you reassess when necessary.

During this stage of caregiving, you will gradually be removing from your loved one's home things like the checkbook and credit cards. But it is important to leave behind items and processes that are still doable for your loved one.

- A delightful example of this was when a caregiver asked her mother to do paper shredding. Her mother was in the Moderate Stage of Alzheimer's disease and could still understand some things about identity theft and the need to shred documents.

Her responsibility in shredding financial documents means she is still participating in her own financial affairs. It isn't necessary to say, "No, Mom, you don't have to shred that; it's just an advertisement that came with the bill." Let her shred it.

In the later stage of the disease, she may have lost all concept of identity theft protection but can still physically carry out the shredding. You can bring to her the things that need shredding. Removal of the shredder would be just one more reminder of what she has lost and doesn't provide her the opportunity to contribute in a way that she is capable of contributing. Maybe you can use a shredder at home. They only cost $25 to $30 at an office supply store.

MODERATE TO SEVERE STAGE

As your loved one moves further into the disease, fewer financial management skills are preserved. Things that she can no longer do become your responsibility or that of someone else in the caregiver "team." The time involved may decrease substantially, because you are able to "just do it" and can tap into your own organizational skills and ways of approaching financial tasks, rather than having to adapt to her traditional way of doing things and supervise her while she is doing them.

Communication takes place at many levels. A person with Alzheimer's disease may not talk at all, but can still mimic actions or can follow directions or can do something that is so overlearned that it is deep in the brain and Alzheimer's disease hasn't gotten to it yet. Go back to your checklist of steps in a task to help you decide if there are any things your loved one can still do.

This is the caregiving phase when you are most likely to need to exercise Power of Attorney (POA) responsibilities. Like every legal tool, the POA contract can be used for good or for evil. You are supposed to make POA decisions with the welfare of your loved one in mind. Reports of abuses by POAs are rampant, but you never hear in the news media about those with POA who are responsibly carrying out the mandate to "act in the best interests of..." No one wants to go to court to ask for guardianship to be established, but if you think that the person with POA is abusing your loved one, a court proceeding may be needed to sort out the issues.

If you are the POA, you will find it worthwhile to keep good records of your dealings with the financial affairs of your loved one. In family meetings, these details will help others in the caregiving "circle" to understand exactly what it is you do and why. These details will also support your use of your loved one's money to reimburse you for expenses you incur on her behalf.

For example, writing down the errands you have done for her can provide the basis for you to fill your gas tank every so often using her credit card. The IRS allows a certain mileage allowance. In lieu of gas money, maybe you pay yourself a mileage allowance.

A side benefit of this recordkeeping is that family members will know that you are providing certain services that they would never have imagined or thought about being necessary.

I remember one Christmas when I shopped for my father's gift list for his grandchildren. It required six different trips to complete the list. Two of those trips were for returns because he didn't care for what I found.

Does your dentist or podiatrist make house calls? If not, then you are probably transporting your father, waiting with him through the appointment, and helping him return home. Did you have to take time away from work to do this? You may want to be compensated for this. Remember, even jury duty merits some compensation ($25 a day in my jurisdiction!)

Finally, all the examples mentioned earlier help you, the caregiver, keep track of expenditures that have occurred during your caregiving days. They will help you and your caregiving team bring closure to financial details of caregiving for a person with Alzheimer's disease or other dementia. The following information is outlined for your quick references when needed.

SIGNS OF FINANCIAL EXPLOITATION

This list comes from many different sources. They represent situations or scenarios in which there is a likelihood of financial exploitation/abuse; keep your eyes and ears open. The perpetrator:

1. Gets access to her checking account.
2. Withholds part of a check cashed for her.
3. Charges an unreasonable amount for basic care services or for shopping.
4. Convinces her to sign over assets.
5. Uses POA to alter her will or borrow money in her name or sell an asset such as her house.
6. Offers to split some found money with her if she puts up some money as a show of good faith.
7. Persuades her to buy an unneeded, valueless, nonexistent, or overpriced product.
8. Persuades her to donate to a bogus charity or invest in a fictitious business.
9. Convinces her to send some money to pay taxes on a sweepstakes "prize".
10. Convinces her that her grandson is in jail in Canada and needs bail money.
11. Stops work in the middle of a repair job and asks for more money.

FINANCIAL RESOURCES FOR CAREGIVERS

Information Sources: AARP, National Alzheimer's Association, state bankers' association, your own bank:

- AARP probably has the most comprehensive set of resources for managing financial affairs of vulnerable adults. It is as close to a "one-stop-shopping" experience as you'll find for information and advocacy. Especially helpful are the resources on insurance and investment products and financial exploitation. You can find such information at the local AARP office, the AARP Internet site, and Borders Bookstores. (A rotator display unit, usually right inside the front door, is stocked with free booklets about many financial issues.)
- Alzheimer's Association local offices also feature many resources for caregivers.
- Every state has a bankers' association, most of which provide exploitation identification training for bank employees.
- Many banks have a "senior services personal banker" kind of position. This employee can discuss with you ways to make financial affairs easier for you to manage with your loved one. One relatively easy step is to set up an electronic automatic bill paying for regular monthly expenses so there is less need for personal intervention of time and resources, and less opportunity for exploitation by someone coming into the home.

Support Entities: Bill paying services, senior companion services, Alzheimer's Association

- AARP Foundation Bill Payer Programs are available in some locations. Volunteers meet with low-income clients one-on-one to help organize bill paying, create a budget, write out checks for the client's signature, balance the client's checkbook, and note issues that are coming up. Volunteers are background screened for credit and criminal activity issues and are supervised. The AARP Foundation provides financial protection of client funds from mistakes by the volunteer. This kind of service is probably best suited for the Early-to-Mild Stage of caregiving.

- Some social service agencies have developed Daily Money Management programs to assist vulnerable elders in protecting their financial security and to serve as a deterrent to financial exploitation. AARP found at least 360 such programs around the country.
- The American Association of Daily Money Managers has a certification program to provide credentials to those who complete the training program.
- Senior companion services (both nonprofit and profit-making businesses) often train their employees in some of the details of helping vulnerable adults cope with routine financial management tasks.
- Caregiver support groups will likely have financial management issues on their agenda. You are all facing similar challenges. Many of you have devised specific ideas for dealing with particular issues that have surfaced. The support group gives a place to ask questions, voice concerns, and contribute your experiences of what has worked and what hasn't worked.
- Law enforcement and government: Adult Protective Services, police, elder abuse hot lines
- Every state has an Adult Protective Services Division. Every call or written inquiry is supposed to be investigated as to its validity. If you think someone is financially abusing a person with Alzheimer's disease or other dementia, this entity can provide an investigation into the charges.
- Likewise, elder abuse reported to the police must be investigated. As many as half of these reports are situations of financial abuse. If you have reason to believe that your loved one is being exploited illegally, call the police.
- Many locales have an Elder Abuse Hot Line. Probably, the easiest way to get information about this is the 211 phone number that is nearly nationwide now. The operators have access to thousands of pieces of referral information to help you find the right place to report an abuse or to ask questions about potential abuses you suspect.

CHAPTER 5

Be Your Own Detective

Patricia R. Callone and Lauren M. Petit

WHAT DOES SHERLOCK HOLMES HAVE TO DO WITH ALZHEIMER'S DISEASE?

Sherlock Holmes is one of the most widely known detectives in literature. Sir Arthur Conan Doyle, the author of the Sherlock Holmes' mysteries, studied to become a medical doctor but found that he didn't want to continue in the profession. Instead Sir Arthur wanted to write. So he used the technique of looking for "clues" and "cues," the skills of observation that he had learned in studying medicine to create the detective Sherlock Holmes.

YOU, the caregiver, are very important to the overall health of your loved one and your family. No one is trained to be a caregiver of a person with dementia. It is an on-the-job training experience. You can learn a lot about Alzheimer's disease and its progression across the brain, but the real part of giving care to your loved one involves detective skills of observation of only one person—your loved one.

As a caregiver, you can become your own detective in understanding your loved one and giving care that is appropriate at each stage of the disease. You are always in the mode of trying to figure out the clues and cues to putting together the pieces of the Alzheimer's caregiving puzzle.

The moment-to-moment clues and cues come from your loved one in words, body movements, smiles, frowns, quietness, anxiety, laughter, crying, and more. Knowing well the particular person for whom you care is the key to being able to give your loving personal touch.

MEET MY LOVED ONE

Like most detectives, you will want to summarize everything you need to know about your loved one and put it in a folder (electronic or paper). Just like the "case files" in a detective series on TV. We suggest you put the information into a booklet form that has specific sections of information easily accessible by you or anyone else who would need access to it. There is a Guide titled "Meet My Loved One" at the end of this chapter (pages 73–85) that can help you make the information attractive and usable for your loved one as well as other family members and friends.

Caregivers who have used this tool, "Meet My Loved One," have found that doing the work of putting together the information has many advantages. Here's why: The booklet helps you keep all the important information about your loved one in one place. It can contain personal and medical information as well as important contacts that you will need as primary caregiver.

The booklet can contain information about the location of your loved one's Living Will, who has been appointed Healthcare Power of Attorney, who has been appointed Durable Power of Attorney for Finances, and so on. (If these decisions have not already been put in place, this is the time to do it.)

Note: Having the Healthcare Power of Attorney in place is actually a gift to you and your family. In the document for healthcare, the person(s) who have Healthcare Power of Attorney should be directed *in writing* (according to an attorney) to share the medical condition of your loved one with others who will be part of your caregiving team. This means that everyone needs to know the wishes of your loved one and abide by them. The Healthcare Power of Attorney has the responsibility to carry out those wishes.

Sadly, sometimes family members, who do not live close to the loved one who has Alzheimer's disease, do not see the changes taking place in the life and care of your loved one. Whoever is Healthcare Power of Attorney needs to have the right to share medical information from medical professionals so all family members can understand decisions that the Healthcare Power of Attorney needs to carry out.

The booklet titled "Meet My Loved One" also has these other advantages. It becomes:

- A history of important moments that your loved one enjoyed in the past.
- An activity for you, your loved one, other family members, and friends to add pictures and stories of celebrations in your family. Pictures of new grandchildren, loved pets, from vacations you take—all are part of "Nurturing What Remains" for your loved one with Alzheimer's disease or other dementia. This ongoing activity will highlight important moments through your years of caregiving.
- If something happens to you and you are not able to continue to care for your loved one, all the information that you have gathered will not be lost. The booklet can be handed to other caregivers, medical professionals, faith leaders, assisted living staff members, and long-term care personnel.
- If your loved one needs the services of hospice, the booklet becomes a wonderful tool for hospice workers and others to know your loved one through the booklet named "Meet My Loved One" _____(Name) by, you (your name) as primary caregiver. Very personal and loving care can be enhanced for hospice personnel as they do their work.

BE YOUR OWN DETECTIVE

Now let's begin the process of "being your own detective." We are beginning to put together the "case file" with information about your loved one. (See the Guide at the end of this chapter.)

1. What personal information do you have about your loved one?

Make a section titled "Personal Information." Here are some suggestions for ways to organize your information:

- Personal Identity—name, address, and so on
- Family and Friends—contact information
- Important Documents—where they can be found

2. What medical information do you have about your loved one?

Make a "Medical Information Section" in your booklet titled "Meet My Loved One." (See the Guide at the end of this chapter.) You may or may not want the help of your loved one while putting this section together. But you need to know about all the frailties of your loved one so that you can give appropriate care. Ask medical professionals for help in understanding your loved one's body. You may want the help of other family members while you put this section together. Answers to these questions and those in the Guide for the booklet will help you gather the information you need. Remember putting this information together is to help you and your loved one enjoy your relationship in caregiving.

- Has your loved one been tested to verify that she/he has dementia?
- Have you received directions about the care of your loved one?
- Does your loved one have trouble hearing, seeing, walking— or other limitations that need to be taken into account in his/her caregiving?
- Is your loved one experiencing depression?
- Does your loved one have a number of medications that could enhance dementia?

Put the answers to these questions in your paper or electronic folder named "Meet My Loved One" so that you can remember these answers as you continue your caregiving over what may be a long period of time. (Update this section of your booklet when more medications are added or some medications are taken away.)

3. What are your loved one's "likes" and "dislikes" and what "environment" does your loved one prefer? (See the Guide at the end of this chapter.)

a. "Likes" and "dislikes"

Record any information that is personal to your loved one that will help you give personalized care. You can put information about these things in the booklet like this:

- Food—different tastes
- Activities—sports, games, gardening, and so on
- Humor
- Pets
- Music
- Schooling
- TV programs
- History—stories of WWI and WWII
- Worship preferences
- Cultural identity
- General health
- General mood
- Special friends
- Work life
- Travel
- Recall three important stories about the person's life
- Ask others how they would describe your loved one in the past
- Add other things that you know are important to your loved one
- Capitalize on your loved one's pleasant memories

Update this section of your booklet as your loved one's preferences for food, activities, and so on change because of the disease progression.

b. "Environment"

Be an intuitive detective and assess the environment in which you care for your loved one. If your loved one likes to be touched, kissed, held, do that often. You can give a sense of security by putting your arms around him/her, by stroking your loved one's hands, by combing your loved one's hair—any way to communicate that you care for your loved one and show that he/she is safe.

Keep the environment free from distractions, pleasant, and safe. You will need to pay attention to changes needed in the environment as the disease progresses. Keep a log of what is safe for your loved one in the room that is "specially" his/hers. Keep a record of what the environment "feels like." Does your loved one like light, color? To sit near a window, to be warm, to be cool? The environment will dictate much of your loved one's moods and can contribute to his/her having feelings of anxiety. (Consult the National Alzheimer's Association and your local Alzheimer's chapter for more information concerning a safe and pleasant environment for your loved one.) Revise this section of the booklet as you become aware of needed changes in the environment for your loved one.

4. What memories does your loved one enjoy?

Make a section titled "Memory Prompts" (see the Guide at the end of this chapter.) This can be fun for you and your loved one as you can discuss "the olden days" that your loved one may remember very clearly. Take some of the years that seem most memorable to your loved one and talk about the cost of a home, a car, gasoline, stamps, milk, bread, who was President of the USA at the time, and so on. (The answers are all in the "Memory Prompts" chart that goes from 1920 to 2009.) In addition, you can talk about the years you have enjoyed together. Record the stories your loved one tells about those years. Did he/she ever have an "ice box"? Does he/she remember when the family got its first TV set?

5. What more information—past and present—can you gather about your loved one?

Make a section titled "More About (name of your loved one)." Nurture his/her mind, body, and spirit. Make this section one that your loved one, you, other family members, and friends can enjoy throughout the caregiving process. This section is for two types of information:

a. Past events that involved your loved one.

Take pictures that are memorable to your loved one and other family members. Ask your loved one to identify (when possible) what is in the picture and ask some questions (when possible) like those under the pictures in the Guide in the back of this chapter. Pictures of your loved one's grandparents, school days, involvement in sports, romance, memories of WWII years, pets, and so on. Or you can tell what you remember about the pictures and the special times that occurred. Your conversations may draw out memories that have been hidden by the disease. Use only pleasurable pictures. If a son or daughter was lost in any war, then don't go to memories or stories of the war. But if a son or daughter served in a war and came home proud of his/her service, then capture those special memories.

b. Current stories/events that involve your loved one—with family, friends, church groups, all social events, and so on.

This section will become more alive and fun as you contribute to it. You can be as creative as you want after you have gathered some personal information, medical information, living preferences, "likes" and "dislikes," and pleasant experiences and stories about your loved one. Its up to you, your family, and friends—caregiving team—to make this booklet come alive and be enjoyable for your loved one, you, and other members of your caregiving team throughout your years of caregiving.

The aforementioned information is given to you to help you become the best detective you can be when it comes to creating the best possible caregiving "partnership" in which you find yourself. If these ideas would not work for you, then find other ways to stimulate the mind, body, and spirit of your loved one so that you can remain a healthy caregiver.

The caregiver's special job is to "Nurture What Remains" in the whole person—mind, body, and spirit. The caregiver looks for "clues" and "cues" from the loved one—in a particular moment— that tells what is needed—in a particular moment—and then acts appropriately. The best things you can give your loved one every day is dignified, appropriate, and safe care.

What does "dignified," "appropriate," and "safe" care mean? The overall understandings of the themes are simple enough to know, but the progression of the disease across the brain defines those themes differently and uniquely according to the special person for whom you care and the stage of Alzheimer's disease he/she is experiencing.

"Dignified care" means to always treat the person as an adult who has lived a life full of experiences that have brought him/her to this moment. Do not talk to your loved one or treat your loved one as if he/she were a child. Don't talk about the disease in front of him/her as if your loved one were not present. Treat your loved one with respect— even though there have been moments through his/her life and your life that have been hurtful. Your loved one probably will not remember those moments and you should try to forgive and forget too.

"Appropriate care" means to find the best way possible to take care of his/her life … no matter what stage. Health professionals, other caregivers, and your local Alzheimer's chapter as well as the National Alzheimer's Association have resources to help you. Appropriate care takes in all the needs of your loved one—mind, body, and spirit. Examples are the following:

When your loved one does not understand what is being said, is it because he/she is hard of hearing? Is it because he/she cannot connect the words in his/her mind to understand the question? Is it both? Your careful observation may lead you to take your loved one to an ear doctor to see if your loved one can be helped to understand what is going on in his/her environment.

Appropriate care means to give your loved one help to understand and do things for himself/herself. Help your loved one continue to be productive and independent in every means possible. Help your loved one take care of his/her body. Don't do it for him/her. If your loved one gets dressed with an orange shirt and purple pants, it doesn't matter. Your loved one got dressed with no one's help! So what if the colors don't match. Who cares? Your loved one accomplished something that is most important to his/her own self-image.

Appropriate care means to talk about the things your loved one expresses. Don't dismiss his/her feelings when your loved one says, "I don't want to have Alzheimer's. There are a lot of other people who deserve this. Not me. Why do I have to have it?" Address his/her comments and emotions the best you can. Discuss with him/her that everybody will become frail with some kind of disease. We don't know why different people have different diseases, but living with our own frailties helps us be kind to others who are suffering in life. By being a good detective in your environment, you will become more and more alert to the little details that will make the environment productive and fulfilling for your loved one and yourself.

"Safe care" means that you and your loved one need to be safe. "Safe" means different things during all stages of Alzheimer's disease. Not letting your loved one cook when he/she no longer understands hot and cold is giving safe care. When the person begins to wander, keeping one safe is getting a wrist-identity band so your loved one can be returned home if/when he/she wanders. In the Severe Stage, it is particularly important for you, as a caregiver, to handle yourself in the following ways. When you approach your loved one:

- Approach your loved one calmly from the front. Do not startle him/her. He/she may not recognize you because of the progression of Alzheimer's disease. Watch your own bodily expressions—face, head, and hands. Make sure you give the message that you are caring and attentive to him/her.
- Begin talking by calling your loved one by his/her name and using a moderate voice that you know he/she can hear.
- Give your loved one your name and identify yourself by wearing a familiar garment or have a familiar object with you.
- Touch your loved one—if he/she likes it. Be attentive to what your loved one is feeling. Go with the feelings of your loved one—not necessarily your own. Learn to live in his/her moment.
- Be prepared to do something that is pleasant and happy for both of you.
- Give your loved one a choice between two things he/she enjoys. Perhaps the booklet that you made with your loved one titled "Meet My Loved One" would be useful in showing him/her the contributions he/she has made in life.
- If your loved one becomes upset, use a distraction of something pleasant like the following: food, music, remembered work the person used to do, pictures of people or things your loved one knows, perhaps a trophy on the table that he/she won, pictures of a loved pet that comforted your loved one in his/her life.
- Make transitions and use distractions in a compassionate way.

ASSESSING THE PHYSICAL AND EMOTIONAL ENVIRONMENTS FOR CAREGIVING

Most caregivers will tell you that the hardest things to handle throughout the disease process are working with the loved one's anxieties and emotions. Here are some emotions you may have to deal with: anger, sadness, frustration, anxiety, irritability, fear, apathy, self-blame, helplessness, and so on. Each caregiver has his/her own ways of giving dignified, appropriate, and safe care—according to the personality of the person with dementia. In the following, we list some common observations by caregivers of persons who have been diagnosed with Alzheimer's disease.

Persons with Alzheimer's disease have told us many things. The book *Speaking Our Minds: Personal Reflections from Individuals with Alzheimer's Disease* by Lisa Snyder is a most useful resource for caregivers of persons with Alzheimer's disease. Ms. Snyder, an experienced social worker, interviewed seven persons with the disease over a period of time. She represents a caring, thoughtful "detective" while interviewing persons in their home environments. Here are some themes she brings to light in her book. Persons with Alzheimer's disease talk about:

- A deep sense of loss. They do not want to be defined as to what they cannot do, but rather by what they can still do (Nurture What Remains).
- Persons feel a sense of isolation. In a familiar setting, sometimes others don't know how to react to them because they have been diagnosed with Alzheimer's disease. Friends and family are sometimes afraid of persons who look or act differently from themselves. Therefore, the person with Alzheimer's disease may shy away from talking with them.
- Each person—in his/her own way—fights to be independent and resents help when he/she does not need it.
- Learning to actively listen to the needs/wants/desires of your loved one is most important.
- Caregivers need to be flexible to adapt to the many changes that will occur in the lives of their loved ones… and their own lives.

The journey of caregiving for your loved one can be very rewarding as you will see in other chapters of this book. Concentrate on ways to take care of YOU, the caregiver, so you can be healthy in mind, body, and spirit during your caregiving days.

Meet My Loved One

— Alexander J. McKenna, M.D. —

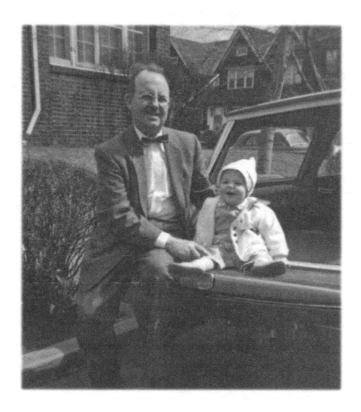

By

Mary T. McKenna

Personal Information

Personal Identity

Legal Name:	Alexander John McKenna, M.D.		
Nickname(s):	Aleck or Allie		
Date of Birth:	October 29, 1906	Place of Birth:	Brooklyn, NY
Home Address:	149 Old County Road, Riverhead, NY 11901		
Home Phone:	516-555-1234	Social Security No. :	XXX-XX-XXXX
Schooling:	Completed High School	Yes_ or No	St. John's Prep
	Completed College:	Yes_ or No	St. John's College
	Completed Professional School:	Yes_ or No	Columbia P&S
Occupation:	Physician	Last employer:	Self-employed
Ethnic/Racial Identity:	Caucasian		
Religious Preference:	Roman Catholic	Parish or home church:	St. Isidore's Church Riverhead, NY
Veteran?	Yes_ or No	Branch of Service:	U. S. Navy

Family and Friends

Primary Caregiver:	Mary T. McKenna		
Relationship to Patient:	Wife		
Address:	149 Old County Road, Riverhead, NY 11901		
Home Phone:	516-555-1234	Cell Phone:	(516) 555-5454
Email Address:	mmm@yyy.org		
Name of Person with Healthcare Power of Attorney:	Same as Primary Caregiver		
Relationship to Patient:	Wife		
Address:	149 Old County Road, Riverhead, NY 11901		
Home Phone:	516-555-1234	Cell Phone:	(516) 555-5454
Email Address:	mmm@yyy.org		

Spouse or Partner:	Mary T. McKenna	
Children and	Daniel McKenna	Janice
Their Spouses:	Albert McKenna	Deidre
	James McKenna	
	Barbara McKenna Dillon	Edmund
	Laura McKenna Small	Chester
Parents:	Alexander and Mary (Meehan) McKenna — both deceased	
Siblings and	Mary McKenna Willy	William Willy
Their Spouses:	John McKenna	

Family and Friends [continued]

Grandchildren:	Linda Dillon		Matthew McKenna
	Alan McKenna		Meredith Small

Other Relatives:	Clare Thorsen (sister-in-law)	*Friends:*	Charles Graves
	Buster Grogan (brother-in-law)		Irky Jussla
	Al Murray (cousin)		Frank Tesoriero
			Bill and Esther Clark
			Rita Hallet

Important Documents and Information

Medicare A:	<u>Yes</u> or No	*Medicare B:*	<u>Yes</u> or No
Other Medical Insurance:	<u>Yes</u> or No	Blue Cross Blue Shield ***Med ID Cards in wallet	
Dental Insurance:	Yes or <u>No</u>		
Vision Insurance:	Yes or <u>No</u>		
Long-Term Care Insurance:	Yes or <u>No</u>		
Medicaid:	Yes or <u>No</u>		

Last Will and Testament:	<u>Yes</u> or No	Safe Deposit Bank @ First National Bank of Riverhead	
Living Will and/or Advanced Directive:	<u>Yes</u> or No	Safe Deposit Bank @ First National Bank of Riverhead	
Durable Power of Attorney for Finances:	<u>Yes</u> or No	Safe Deposit Bank @ First National Bank of Riverhead	
Driver's License	<u>Yes</u> or No	License in wallet	
Passport	<u>Yes</u> or No	Safe Deposit Bank @ First National Bank of Riverhead	

Current Photo:

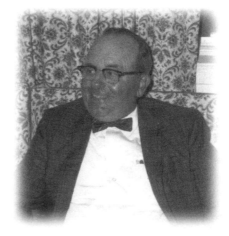

Medical Information

Doctor(s): *(with specialty)*	John B. Smith, M.D. 222 Highway A Riverhead, NY 11901	(516) 555-3333	Internist
	William Q. Jones, M.D. 135 Main Street, Suite B Riverhead, NY 11901	(516) 555-4444	Cardiologist
	Seymor Senick, D.D.S 3705 East 37th Street Riverhead, NY 11901	(516) 555-7777	Dentist
	Raymond Inman, M.D. 135 Main Street, Suite K Riverhead, NY 11901	(516) 555-6666	Ophthalmologist

Medical Concerns:
Cardiovascular disease
Dementia
Varicose veins
Thyroid disease

Allergies:
Penicillin
Almonds

Medications: Plavix XXmg (every 12 hours)
(with dosage) Synthroid

Dietary Restrictions:	Low sodium Low fat	*Dietary Preferences:*	(YES) ice cream (NO) peas
Physical Activity *Requirements:*	Walk 15 minutes every day	*Physical Activity* *Restrictions:*	No heavy lifting

Wheelchair:	Yes or <u>No</u>	*Walker:*	<u>Yes</u> or No
Eye glasses?	<u>Yes</u> or No	*Eye Glass Prescription:*	2.25 readers
Dentures?	<u>Yes</u> or No	*Hearing Aid:*	Yes or <u>No</u>
Prosthetic?	Yes or <u>No</u>	*Describe:*	

Environment/Living Space

Likes

Green plants
Classical music
Westerns on TV
Back rubs
Walks outside
Dogs
Fishing and hunting

Charles Dickens novels
Warm temperatures and sunshine
Taking naps
The color blue
Baseball, especially the Dodgers
Brooklyn
A Manhattan after dinner
Bow ties

Dislikes

Noisy children
Cats
Traffic
Being rushed
The color red
The NY Yankees
Massachusetts
In-laws

Other important information to help caregivers give dignified, appropriate and safe care to your loved one [date the information as you enter it].

Memory Prompts

	1920	1930	1940	1950	1960
House	$6,296.00	$7,146.00	$3,925.00	$8,450.00	$12,675.00
Car	$525.00	$610.00	$850.00	$1,511.00	$26,100.00
Gasoline	13¢/gallon	10¢/gallon	11¢/gallon	17¢/gallon	25¢/gallon
Stamps	2¢ each	2¢ each	3¢ each	3¢ each	4¢ each
Milk	29¢/gallon	56¢/gallon	51¢/gallon	84¢/gallon	1.04¢/gallon
Bread	15¢/loaf	9¢/loaf	8¢/loaf	17¢/loaf	20¢/loaf
Life Expectancy	54.1 years	59.7 years	62.9 years	68.2 years	69.7 years
U.S. President	Woodrow Wilson	Herbert Hoover	Franklin D. Roosevelt	Harry Truman	Dwight D. Eisenhower
Memory Prompts	U.S. Post Office prohibits children being sent via Parcel Post.	Pluto, the 9th planet in our solar system, is discovered.	Winston Churchill becomes Prime Minister of Great Britain.	Nat King Cole croons about "Mona Lisa."	CIA pilot Gary Powers is shot down over Soviet Union.
	Gaston Chevrolet wins the Indianapolis 500.	Duke Ellington's big hit is "Three Little Words."	Dr. Charles Drew opens the 1st U.S. blood bank.	The Brinks Robbery takes place in Boston.	Xerox unveils the 1st commercial copy machine.
	The 19th Amendment grants women the right to vote in U.S. elections.	"All Quiet on the Western Front" wins the Academy Award.	The Heisman Trophy goes to Tom Harmon of the University of Michigan.	Truman orders federal troops to take control of U.S. railroads to prevent a strike.	Southern senators filibuster 83 hours in opposition to Civil Rights legislation.
	U.S. rejects the League of Nations.	"The Lone Ranger" airs on the radio.	The World's Fair reopens in NYC.	North Korea invades South Korea.	The Andy Griffith Show is a TV hit.
	Boston's WGI broadcasts 1st scheduled radio programming.	The 1st red and green traffic lights are installed in NYC.	The movie "Rebecca" wins the Academy Award for Best Picture.	The FBI begins publicizing its "10 Most Wanted Criminals" List.	Chubby Checker introduces "The Twist."
	Prohibition goes into effect.	Donald Duck makes his big screen debut.	The 1st televised basketball game: Fordham 37, Pitt 50.	Oklahoma wins the College Football Championship.	The 1st weather satellite is launched.
	Al Jolson sings "Swanee."	Bobby Jones wins the U.S. Open.	FDR is elected to a 3rd term as U.S. President.	The first organ transplant is performed.	Arnold Palmer wins the U.S. Open.

Compiled by Lauren M. Petit, Holy Cow! Word Processing, using *Remember When…A Nostalgic Look Back in Time* [Seek Publishing] and other resources.

Memory Prompts
[continued]

1970	1980	1990	2000	2009	
$23,400.00	$68,714.00	$123,000.00	$134,150.00	$208,600.00	House
$3,979.00	$7,201.00	$16,012.00	$24,750.00	$26,300.00	Car
37¢/gallon	$1.15/gallon	$1.34/gallon	$1.95/gallon	$2.67/gallon	Gasoline
6¢ each	15¢ each	25¢ each	33¢ each	44¢ each	Stamps
1.32¢/gallon	2.02¢/gallon	2.78¢/gallon	$2.99/gallon	$3.39/gallon	Milk
24¢/loaf	51¢/loaf	70¢/loaf	$1.72/loaf	$1.60/loaf	Bread
70.8 years	73.7 years	75.4 years	76.9 years	78.4 years	Life Expectancy
Richard Nixon	Jimmy Carter	George H. W. Bush	Bill Clinton	Barack Obama	U.S. President
The U.S. voting age is lowered from 21 to 18.	CNN begins broadcasting the 1st 24-hour cable news.	San Francisco 49ers win the Super Bowl.	Lance Armstrong wins the "Tour de France" … again.	The 1st African-American president takes office.	Memory Prompts
Ray Stevens sings "Everything is Beautiful."	30% of U.S. auto sales are of imports.	East and West Germany are reunited.	The Yankees win their 26th World Series title.	LA Lakers win their 15th NBA championship.	
The crew of Apollo 13 survives a near-fatal explosion while en route to the moon.	Tip O'Neill is Speaker of the House of Representatives.	The Hubble Space Telescope is placed in orbit by the Space Shuttle Discovery.	Two genetics research teams complete mapping the human genome.	The 1st cases of H1N1 flu virus are diagnosed in Mexico.	
Hawaii Five-O airs on CBS.	Mount Saint Helens erupts.	Iraqi forces invade Kuwait.	CBS's "Survivor" is a summer smash.	Michael Jackson, "King of Pop," dies.	
Nebraska, Texas, and Ohio State are all College Football Champions.	The U.S. boycotts the Moscow Olympics.	Mikhail Gorbachev wins the Nobel Peace Prize.	Charles Schulz, creator of the Peanuts comic strip, dies.	The People's Republic of China celebrates its 60th Anniversary.	
The U.S. military invades Laos and Cambodia.	Philadelphia Phillies win the World Series.	Nelson Mandela is released from prison.	Sidney, Australia hosts the Summer Olympics.	NBC's "Saturday Night Live" begins its 35th season.	
The World Trade Center opened in NYC.	"The Love Boat" is a popular TV show.	Jim Henson, founder of the Muppets, dies.	Y2K is a non-event.	UNESCO launches The World Digital Library.	

Compiled by Lauren M. Petit, Holy Cow! Word Processing, using *Remember When…A Nostalgic Look Back in Time* [Seek Publishing] and other resources.

More About Aleck McKenna

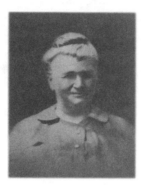 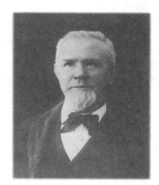

Here are pictures of your grandparents, Peter and Ellen (Mahern) Brenner.

- Both of your grandparents were born in Ireland; they came to the United States in the 1870s. Do you recall any stories they may have told you about "the Old Country" and about their arrival in America?

- Your grandparents were very much a part of your life when you were growing up. They always lived nearby ... and for a time, you actually lived with them ... in one of the three-story walk-ups on Gold Street and North Oxford Street in Brooklyn. Today, that area is called Vinegar Hill, but back when you were small it had another name. What did you call that part of Brooklyn?

- Did you enjoy living with your grandparents? In the pictures, they look like very kind, caring people. What can you tell me about them? As their firstborn grandchild, how did they make you feel special?

- About the time these pictures were taken, your grandfather was working as a night watchman at the nearby gas plant. Did you ever visit him there? Your grandmother ran a soup kitchen in her home for the workers at the nearby Brooklyn Navy Yard. You've said in the past she was an excellent cook. What were your favorite meals that she cooked?

- What is a favorite memory of your grandparents?

To Stimulate Memories of Your School Days

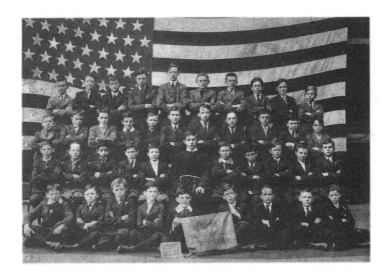

Here is a picture of your seventh grade class at Sacred Heart School in Brooklyn.

- Can you pick out where you are seated? [Hint: you are in the front row, second from the left].

- You don't seem very happy in the picture, but then most of the boys seem rather glum sitting there with their arms folded tight? Do you know why everyone looked so serious?

- This was a Catholic parochial school. What religious order ran the school? Was the brother seated in the middle of the picture your teacher? He doesn't seem much older than you and your classmates. Do you know anything about that young man? Was he a good teacher? Strict? Fair?

- Who in the picture were your friends? Did you have a best friend?

- What did you like best about school? What is a favorite memory from your school days?

To Stimulate Memories of Your Favorite Sports

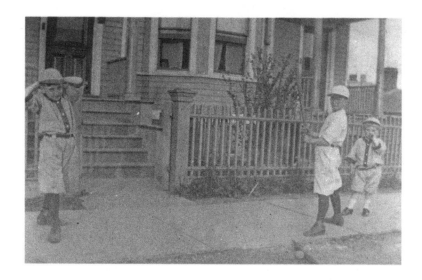

Here is a picture of you playing baseball with friends from your neighborhood.

- You've always loved baseball, even when you were a little boy. Can you name the two other boys and where they lived? Whose house is that in the background?

- You are wearing a uniform in the picture. What was the name of your team? Was there a sandlot or field nearby where you could play, or did you just play in the street?

- As a Brooklyn boy, what teams did you root for? I remember you as being a diehard Dodgers fan even after they moved to California. When did you first become a Dodgers fan?

- Who was your favorite Dodger baseball player?

- Why did Dodgers fans hate the New York Yankees so much? Did you ever cheer for the Yankees?

- What is a favorite memory involving baseball?

To Stimulate Memories of Past Romances

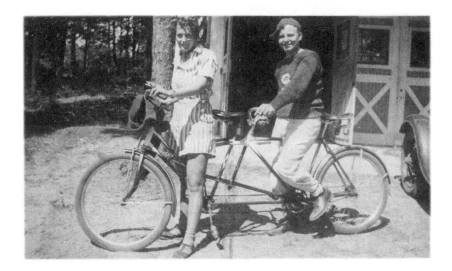

Here is a picture of your wife Mary (Craig) and you when you were dating.

- Do you remember anything about this particular day? Where was this picture taken? Did Marion and you often go bicycle riding? What other sort of fun things did you do when you were dating?

- When you two met, Mary was a nursing student at St. Mary's Hospital in Brooklyn, and you were an intern there. What was Mary like when you first met her? How was she different than the other nursing students?

- Did it matter that you were eight years older than Mary was? Was it love at first sight?

- In this picture, both you and Mary are smoking cigarettes. When did you first start smoking, and how long did you continue to smoke?

- What is a favorite memory about dating Mary?

To Stimulate Memories of the War Years

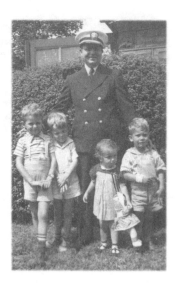

Here is a picture of you in your Navy uniform with your four small children.

- At the beginning of World War II, you were thirty-five years old, a father with four children, and busy with a medical practice. And yet you enlisted in the Navy rather than wait to be drafted. Why did you pick the Navy?

- How did you feel wearing that uniform? How did your family feel about you volunteering for military service? Were they proud, frightened, enthused? Did other colleagues enlist as well?

- As a doctor, your services were much needed by the Navy during the war. You were first stationed to a Marine camp in North Carolina. How would you describe your time there?

- Later in the war, you were reassigned to a posting in Manhattan ... much closer to Brooklyn! How did it feel to be able to come home every night to your family?

- How did your military service change your life? Do you feel you are a stronger person for having lived through that period?

- What is your strongest memory from your Navy days?

To Stimulate Memories of Your Favorite Pets

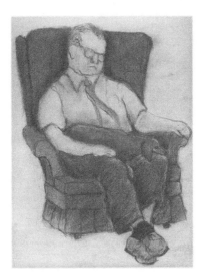

Here is a drawing of you with your dachshund Otto.

- You've always loved dogs ...even as a little boy. What is it about dogs that you like so much?

- Can you remember any of your dogs? In the 1950s, you had a black cocker spaniel named Jinx. Mom always said he was a real troublemaker. What sort of mischief did he get into?

- When I was six years old, you bought me a dachshund as a Christmas present. We named him Otto. Even though he was supposed to be my dog, Otto really was yours. What was it about Otto that you loved so much?

- Otto and you were very set in your ways. Every evening, after your last patient left the office, you two would go for a walk. Where did you walk? Who did you meet along the way?

- After dinner, you would put on the TV, sit in your favorite chair with Otto on your lap, and go to sleep. What is a favorite memory of Otto?

The Alzheimer's Caregiving Puzzle: Taking Care of YOU!

CHAPTER 6

Five Healthy Caregiving Practices

Patricia R. Callone

Life has invited you to become a caregiver of a person with Alzheimer's disease or other dementia. It doesn't matter what circumstances have occurred to name you a "caregiver." You may be a son, daughter, grandson, granddaughter, spouse, son-in-law, daughter-in-law, grandchild, niece, nephew, or friend. Although this may be a scary time for you, it is also a special and unique time in your life. You are being presented with many opportunities for self-growth if you take the time to care for yourself. As a result of this experience, your family may become much closer and realize the blessings you have in each other.

You are not alone. In the United States, about 60 percent of family and other unpaid caregivers are women. Because Alzheimer's disease usually progresses slowly, most caregivers spend many years in the caregiving process at the same time they manage other responsible roles in their lives—such as parenting children; working for pay outside the home; living in partnership with a spouse or other loved ones; helping with the care of grandchildren, and so on.

THE ROLE OF "CAREGIVER" HAS EXPANDED OVER THE YEARS

Old Model: When I was in high school, I worked part-time in a hospital where my mom worked in the health insurance area. In the 1950s and 1960s, a patient could come into the hospital, have surgery, and if the patient had two insurance policies, they would both pay for the operation. The patient could stay as many as 5 days or more and be treated by a team of healthcare professionals in the hospital who came to know the uniqueness of each patient. Then, when the patient returned home, the loved one could be cared for by family members who knew pretty much what their roles were in the patient's healing process. At that time, many family caregivers did not work outside the home.

Today's Model: In 2010, because of payment regulations for healthcare in the United States, doctors generally can spend from 15 to 20 minutes with the patient at the doctor's office. (My experience with my husband, who has had many surgeries and takes 21 pills a day, is the following: the time with the doctor is generally used for a brief examination, discussion of why the patient is there, and ends with a prescription for medication or further tests to be done on the patient. If surgery has to be done, the stay in the hospital is minimal. When the patient is dismissed, caregivers need to assume caregiving responsibilities for which they are not trained.)

If you are a caregiver to someone who has Alzheimer's disease or other dementia and your loved one needs other medical attention, such as a surgery, management of diabetes, and so on, YOU become the focal point for your loved one's care. YOU—for the sake of your loved one—interact with all of the following: medical doctors, nurses, physical therapists, occupational therapists, pharmacists, dentists, doctors for eyes and ears, and representatives from community services agencies, your faith community, assisted living and long-term care facilities, and possibly hospice. In summary, YOU are the one who manages all the care of your loved one. In addition, somewhere in the caregiving process YOU will become involved with the family finances to provide ongoing care. YOU become the advocate for the dignified, appropriate, and safe care of your loved one.

Generally, your loved one—because of the dementia—will not remember or understand the directions or advice that is being given. YOU become the "interpreter" of all the messages given about care for your loved one. YOU interpret messages from one doctor to another or changes in medication to other persons who are helping you give care. YOU are a very important part of the caregiving team—because you are the one who gives care 24/7. YOU are the one who instinctively knows when change is taking place and transitions need to be made.

The very difficult role for the caregiver is to try to balance all the messages from healthcare professionals so you can give dignified, appropriate, and safe care to your loved one AND remain healthy and energetic in your own life. You may ask, "Is that really possible?" The answer is, "Yes," with the wisdom and guidance from other caregivers and healthcare professionals.

The areas most caregivers need assistance with for themselves are these: ways to alleviate stress; ways to take time for themselves and other family members; ways to manage the financial burden, and ways to continue to be productive and active members in their communities. Caring for a person with Alzheimer's disease and other dementia is like trying to put together the pieces of a puzzle. You know the pieces will make a full picture, but where to put the pieces and when to put them in is the real task. In the caregiving puzzle, sometimes you cannot even imagine what the picture is supposed to look like. Our goal is to help you, the caregiver, put together a puzzle that has this end result:

- A beautiful picture of your loved one receiving dignified, appropriate, and safe care
- You living a meaningful and healthy life

Some people have been known to become exhausted while trying to do all the caregiving and at the same time they carry on all the other responsibilities of work and family. The stresses on your mind and body can injure your own health and sometimes cause your own death before the death of the person for whom you care. We do not want that to happen to you.

Keep in mind you already know quite a bit about caregiving. You have had a lifetime of experiences that shape your attitudes about it. You have watched other members of your family care for those who have been frail or ill. Perhaps you watched your mother care for her mother or your father care for his parents. You already have garnered some information from books, movies, TV. You have witnessed the joys and sorrows of caregiving because life involves all of us in caregiving responsibilities and duties.

However, you may not feel you have the skills you need to manage full-time caregiving for a person with dementia. You need to be open to listening to the guidance of healthcare professionals, other people in your situation, and most importantly—listen to the "needs" and "wants" of your loved one. There is a difference between the "needs" of your loved one—which imply dignified, appropriate, and safe care—and the "wants" of your loved one—which imply desires that may or may not be able to be fulfilled.

In this part of the book, we have outlined some ways to help you keep yourself healthy in mind, body, and spirit through your caregiving days. We call them "Five Healthy Caregiving Practices."

1. Keep focused on your goals.
2. Understand yourself as a caregiver. Your needs will change.
3. Try to understand your loved one. Nurture what your loved one can still do.
4. Keep communication open at all times.
5. Strengthen your spiritual base.

1. Keep focused on your goals.
- To give dignified, appropriate, and safe care to your loved one throughout the progression of the disease
- To enrich your own life (mind, body, spirit) throughout the caregiving process

What do you think about those two goals? Do those goals fit what you want to happen as you give care to your loved one? Modify these goals for yourself if they don't fit you. State what you want to be the end result of your caregiving days.

2. Understand yourself as a caregiver. Your needs will change.

You will want to evaluate your personal strengths and weaknesses as a caregiver throughout the disease process. Your strengths and weaknesses will evolve over time. If you are the primary caregiver, now is the time for you to reflect on the particular strengths and weaknesses you have as a caregiver. Some people cannot do this as well as others. It is better for you, the person with dementia, and other family members to be honest about what strengths and weaknesses you have and in what caregiving situations you will need help. No one person can be expected to take care of all the responsibilities of caring for a person with dementia or Alzheimer's.

This should be a team effort throughout the disease process. You will want to stay connected to your life resources. If you are the primary caregiver for a loved one who has dementia, you become the "Coach" of all possible team members. Your numerous life resources and some of your team members are these: other family members, other caregivers, medical professionals, friends and neighbors, your faith community, your local Alzheimer's chapter, and National Alzheimer's Association (www.alz.org).

The caregiving team members—whether near or far away—can contribute something. Those not involved in personal caregiving may be able to help in the following ways:

- Contribute money to help purchase items or clothes needed for the loved one
- Drive the loved one to get groceries, go to church, go to doctors' visits
- Visit the loved one so the primary caregiver can get away for 2 to 3 hours
- Arrange to have meals made for you, your family, and your loved one with dementia
- Provide emotional support (caregiving buddy) for the primary caregiver

You won't need your team resources all the time, but you need to keep in mind the fact that you cannot do it all alone. You need to use the resources available to you when the demands of caregiving increase.

You will need to learn to balance your life with your caregiving duties. You probably have a number of other roles and responsibilities such as being a husband, wife, mother, father, daughter, son, employee, volunteer, and so on. Learn to say, "I need help with this now." Or to say, "I can't do this anymore, but I can do that..."

You can expect changes and transitions for yourself throughout the disease process. Your loved one will realize increasingly that he/she cannot do the things he/she used to do. The person doesn't want to admit something is changing in his/her abilities to control his/her own life. Your loved one may be depressed and angry that this is happening not only to him/her but also to you and your family.

The transitions from one caregiving stage to the next will take more time and energy from you and your team. You will need to look for "clues" and "cues" to move from one stage to the next.

Your attitude toward giving care is very important. Your attitude affects "how" you give care and react to your loved one. Your attitude is communicated by your words, actions, moods, body language, and so on. Your loved one intuitively knows how you feel about him/her by what is picked up by your loved one's senses. If you are stressed or hurried or happy and relaxed, your mind, body, and spirit can be communicated to your loved one who has dementia. Your loved one knows the environment mostly through his/her senses.

Try to be mindful of the ways in which you are growing as a caregiver. You will have opportunities to learn how to be more self-disciplined and compassionate. You will have times when you learn to evaluate what is important and what is not important to get done. You will have times that you realize that pleasing your loved one is much more important than pleasing yourself. Learn to live in your loved one's moment. Throughout your caregiving days you will have time to reflect on the meaning of your own life as well as the lives of others. You can see more clearly what is important and what is not.

It is important to try to find humor in life's situations. There are good examples in the chapters in the rest of this book that show how "humor" can be a lifesaver for everyone involved. You can find humor as you learn to live with your own frailties and the frailties of others as you give care to others.

Create a team of caregivers for your loved one and yourself. You and your team of caregivers can become great friends as you find out the new talents and humor of other team members. Everyone can become closer to your loved one and your whole family because you have shared these moments that will be remembered in the future. You can then become someone who can assist your friends and neighbors who may become involved in caring for a loved one with dementia in their own families.

What do you think are your strengths in caregiving? What are your weaknesses? Who do you think could be part of your caregiving team? For your loved one? For yourself? If you like to journal, begin now to journal about the above comments. Write the date on the sheet so when you look back a year from now, you can review the changes that have taken place in yourself as caregiver.

3. **Try to understand your loved one. Nurture what your loved one can still do.**

Help your loved one be in charge of his/her responsibilities as long as possible. Like most of us, your loved one does not want to become dependent on anyone. People always want to be in control of their own lives. We want to be self-sufficient. Our American culture has taught us that. That doesn't change for the person with dementia. Your loved one would probably prefer to be giving care rather than receiving care.

It is important to treat your loved one as an adult with likes and dislikes and a personal history that should be respected. Look for clues that show you the person needs more help than before. If the person seems stuck or not to know what to do next, prompt the person so he/she can move forward with your help. There are many ways to "prompt" your loved one to do things for himself/herself—whether engaging in fun activities, eating, taking care of personal needs. Just remember that you want to prompt your loved one to do the activity himself/herself, with your assistance, not your control.

Remember to take time for rest, for stimulation, and for taking care of your loved one's personal needs as well as your own. Help your loved one stay connected socially to family, friends, members of his/her faith community, and participation in meaningful cultural activities.

Think about the ways in which your loved one can be stimulated, safe, and feel a sense of purpose. Review again the information you gathered for the booklet titled "Meet My Loved One." Try to make all situations as pleasant as possible. Avoid stressful situations for yourself and your loved one. You can keep a daily rhythm that your loved one and you can depend on and enjoy. Is there something special that you can do together that is special to do on weekends? Certain days of the week?

4. Keep communication open at all times.

Look for clues to transitions that are taking place. Let your loved one talk about his/her feelings. You and other family members should be honest about how you feel also. Concentrate on what your loved one can still do. Many successful caregiving situations begin with OPENLY talking about the changes occurring in everyone's lives.

Early in the disease progression, comments from the person who is diagnosed with dementia may be:

- This isn't what I expected. All our lives we have delayed having "fun" until our children were raised... now... I'm not so sure we can do that now.
- I don't like this! I can't do things like I used to do.
- There isn't anything wrong with me! I don't want to be dependent on anyone.

Your comments and those of other family members who are caregiving may be:

- I don't know what to do, but I'll take time to learn.
- I am afraid I won't be a good enough caregiver.
- I'm not the right person to give care to Mom/Dad/Aunt Ethel/ Uncle Don... maybe someone else.
- I am going to need help because I have responsibilities other than being a caregiver.

Be open and honest with all family members about the physical and mental condition of your loved one. Sometimes relatives near and far can't see the changes that are taking place in your loved one. When family members don't see the changes, they can think you might be exaggerating some of your loved one's behaviors. Ask family members to meet with you, the doctor, and your loved one so that everyone understands how the disease is affecting your family.

When you need help because of your own physical well-being, say so. Have a plan in mind that will assist you and your loved one. When you need assistance daily, ask for it. Talk with your local Alzheimer's chapter and see if there are ways in which you can receive "respite care."

Meaningful, honest conversations can help build trust, which makes a strong, healthy base for caregiving. It doesn't matter what the feelings are. Try to separate facts from feelings. Talking honestly about each person's feelings—for the person with the disease, the caregiver, family members, and health professionals—is important.

This communication can clear the air and relieve stress for all involved.

5. Strengthen your spiritual base.

There are new studies about resilient people that tell us that resilient people call on their inner strength and use networks of resources to keep moving forward. They have the capacity to adjust their future expectations to fit their "new life reality"—whether it is the loss of a job or loved one, a diagnosis of a disease, or some financial crisis.

In the article "The Secrets of Resilient People" by Beth Howard (AARP, November/December 2009), the author quotes Sam Goldstein, a psychologist at the University of Utah, "Like almost any behavior, resilience can be learned."

Research shows that resilient people share some common qualities—ones you can cultivate to master many crises. They stay connected; are optimistic, spiritual, playful; give back; pick their battles; stay healthy; and find the silver lining.

Research also shows that physical exercise can help clear the mind and produce healthy bodies. Exercise should fit you and your body. Take into account your age and bodily health. Sometimes yoga and similar practices work best for relieving stress. Pick what fits you—mind, body, and spirit—and take time to refresh your spirit.

If you find wisdom in the aforementioned information, you can choose to practice some of those qualities as caregiving situations present themselves to you. Prayer and reflection about life as it presents itself to you are powerful tools for "resilience." Take time for silence by turning off the radio in the car or turning off the TV when you have already heard the news once. Take a walk over the noon hour at work; read inspiring material; listen to music that gives you enjoyment; walk the dog into nature areas that show the change of seasons, and so on.

If you and your loved one believe in life after death, here is an image that can comfort you. There are two passages that each individual's spirit makes:

1. There is the passage from the womb to life on earth. There is usually a 9 month period of preparation and then birthing into a new kind of life.

2. Then there is the passage from earthly life into a spiritual world. There is also a preparation for this new birth.

Both passages entail transitions that are painful, but result in new life in a different way.

If you are journaling, you may want to write what you think are some of the ways that bring your spirit refreshment. Is it quiet time alone? Prayer alone or with others? Exercise—swimming, walking? Playing music yourself or listening to others play? Having a cup of coffee and good conversation with a long-time friend? Whatever it is, make time for you to be nourished. This should be as much a part of your caregiving day as all the other responsibilities you have. If you do not take time for yourself to be refreshed in spirit, you will not be able to sustain your health during this time of your life.

The needs of caregivers of persons with Alzheimer's disease and other dementia evolve over time. Just as your loved one will go through stages of the disease, so you will go through different stages of caregiving. We believe the "Five Healthy Caregiving Practices" we have just discussed can help create the overall picture for the Alzheimer's Caregiving puzzle that addresses you and your growth as you give care to your loved one who has Alzheimer's disease or other dementia.

If you find these five caregiving practices helpful, then post them where you can review them daily. Modify these goals using your own words so they become helpful reminders for YOU:

1. Keep focused on your two main goals:
   - To give dignified, safe, and appropriate care to your loved one throughout the progression of the disease
   - To enrich your own life (mind, body, spirit) throughout the caregiving process
2. Understand yourself as a "caregiver." Your needs will change. Evaluate your personal strengths and weaknesses as a caregiver. Again, this should be a team effort throughout the disease process. Stay connected to your life's resources, and learn to balance the demands of your life with your caregiving duties. Expect changes and transitions and monitor your attitude about caregiving. Be mindful of the ways in which you yourself are growing.

3. Try to understand your loved one. Nurture what he/she can still do. Help your loved one be in charge of his/her life and responsibilities as long as possible. Treat your loved one as an experienced adult who has managed to live through many changing times in his/her life. Look for clues of anxiety that show your loved one needs help. Concentrate on the good times and memories of the past that continue to give your loved one's life meaning. Keep a daily rhythm that your loved one enjoys and does not create arguments. Be mindful of the ways in which your loved one can be stimulated, safe, and feel a sense of accomplishment.

4. Keep communication open all the time. Honest, meaningful communication can help build trust which makes a strong, healthy base for caregiving.

5. Strengthen your spiritual base. Engage in things that lift your spirits and make you happy. Discipline yourself to stay connected with your faith, community, and your friends—all who can be supportive and important nourishment for you.

CHAPTER 7

Stages of Caregiving: What Caregivers Need at Each Stage

Patricia R. Callone

THE PRE-ALZHEIMER'S STAGE OF CAREGIVING: WHAT DO CAREGIVERS NEED?

Many former caregivers say the two most necessary qualities for caregivers to cultivate are having a sense of humor and patience. Caregivers—you and others—need to remember that persons with Alzheimer's disease cannot control how the disease affects them. But you can control how you relate to your loved ones.

Just as it is useful to talk about the "stages of Alzheimer's disease" across the brain and the care of persons with dementia during those stages, it is important to talk about the "stages of caregiving" that caregivers go through as their loved ones transition through the progression of their disease. Just as the "stages of Alzheimer's disease" are not clearly defined, so neither are the "stages of caregiving" clearly defined. Everything remains a "puzzle." The puzzle needs to be put together thoughtfully and carefully so that both you, as the caregiver, and your loved one can have lives full of meaning and happiness.

We understand there is no one perfect way to give care, but we also have learned from others that some ways work better than others. This chapter is written to help you keep healthy while caregiving. We will be discussing ways to keep yourself healthy—mind, body, and spirit—so that you can more easily handle the various changes in your loved one who has Alzheimer's disease.

Remember that each person experiences Alzheimer's disease uniquely. Thus, each caregiver experiences caregiving uniquely.

Your own personality, passions, "likes" and "dislikes," strengths and weaknesses play a part in keeping yourself healthy as well as keeping your loved one as healthy as possible. It is a "partnership" that you create during this process. You have your contributions to make to the partnership and your loved one has his/her contributions to make to the "caregiving partnership."

Before you or other family members recognize clues that something may be wrong with your loved one's thinking ability to care for himself/herself, you may be giving care to your loved one in other ways. You may have helped your loved one purchase glasses or a hearing aid, or given care after a knee surgery. The point is that before diagnosis your loved one is functioning quite well and living life as best he/she can—even with physical frailties. You and other family members may attribute "old age" to behaviors that interfere with your loved one's ability to take care of himself/herself.

About Your Loved One

When you do recognize that some cognitive abilities are changing and your loved one cannot handle caring for himself/herself as well as in the past, then you need a medical professional to examine your loved one. If/when your loved one receives a diagnosis of Alzheimer's disease or other dementia, then think back to this stage—the Pre-Alzheimer's Stage—and recall what strengths and weaknesses he/she had then.

Understanding your loved one's sense of purpose, passions, energy for life, "likes" and "dislikes," what stimulates him/her intellectually, emotionally, socially, spiritually, aesthetically, and physically in the Pre-Alzheimer's Stage—gives you the BASE from which to give person-centered care to your loved one

The following chart was developed by a caregiver who took care of three loved ones in her family over a period of 18 years (Figure 7.1). She chose these five functions to visually represent for herself and her family what was going on as Alzheimer's disease progressed in the lives of her loved ones: Memory, Language, Complex Tasks, Social Skills, and Senses.

Begin to visually develop the base of information about your loved one that will help you throughout your caregiving days, months, and years. Make a simple chart about your loved one similar

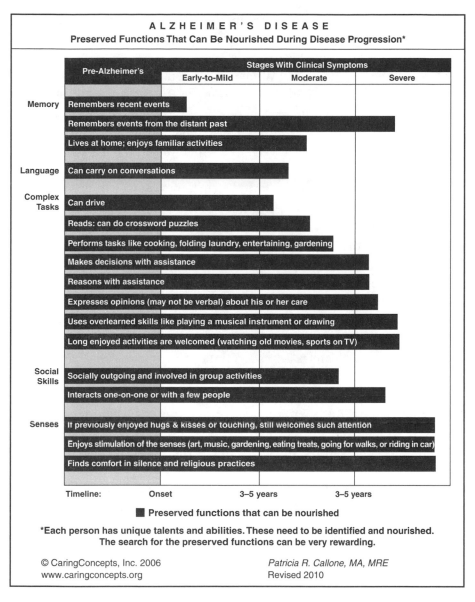

Figure 7.1   A Caregiver's Perspectives, Pre-Alzheimer's.

to Figure 7.1. Title the first heading at the top "Pre-Alzheimer's Disease." Review how your loved one's life has unfolded. Review the information you may have compiled for the "Meet My Loved One" booklet developed in the "Be Your Own Detective" chapter. In this Pre-Alzheimer's Stage, your loved one could hold a job, take care of him/herself, be a productive member of the community, take care of others, and so on. Under the top heading of "Pre-Alzheimer's" fill in answers under the side headings to these:

Referring to "Memory": What have been your loved one's purposes and passions for life? What does he/she still love to do? Do friends come to visit and talk about the "old days" and play music that they danced to as they grew up? Name and list those strengths that have to do with your loved one's "memory."

Referring to "Language": What personality traits have belonged to your loved one? Always good with language? Carried on long conversations? Completed high school, college, graduate education, and more? Has your loved one been employed to use language skills? Educator? Salesperson? Or has he/she worked more with his/her hands and body? A factory worker? Mechanic? Farmer? Whatever have been the strengths of your loved one generally will remain strong throughout the Early-to-Mild Stage and most of the Moderate Stage. Name and list those strengths that have to do with your loved one's "language skills."

Referring to "Complex Tasks": What complex tasks has your loved one enjoyed during his/her lifetime? Has he/she enjoyed physical stimulation in sports? Intellectual stimulation and involvement with music, art, quilting? Enjoyed playing cards, dominos, chess? Driving? Cooking? Crossword puzzles? Taking care of the family finances? Name and list those strengths that have to do with "complex tasks."

Referring to "Social Skills": What does your loved one prefer? Is he/she social, outgoing? Or is he/she more shy and happy to be content at home with a few visitors or family members? What are his/her particular "likes" and "dislikes"? Name and list those strengths that have to do with "social skills."

Referring to "Senses": What senses are still most healthy for your loved one? Is there a need for hearing aids or new glasses? Sometimes hearing is the hardest for everyone to deal with because the person with Alzheimer's disease may not believe he/she has a need for a hearing aid. But you and other family members may have a difficult time getting your loved one's attention. In addition, sometimes your loved one cannot understand what is being said. It can be a combination of "not being able to put together thoughts to understand" and "the ear not working properly to be able to hear." Be sure to face your loved one when talking with him/her and ask others to learn to do this too. Taking steps to get hearing tests can result in relief for all and better communication for everyone.

What other senses are strong and enjoyable for your loved one to use? Enjoys special foods? Enjoys being with and touching special pets? Enjoys art, music, and so on? Name and list as much information about the senses as you can.

Remember your loved one will continue to live and enjoy life through the stimulation of his/her senses all the rest of his/her life. Capitalize on stimulating the senses throughout your loved one's life while being physically and mentally stimulated as well as when your loved one is at rest. Doing this will bring contentment to your loved one and you too. Keep in mind that you are "partners in caregiving" during this Pre-Alzheimer's stage. Having answered these questions while making a chart about your loved one, you now have a firm base from which to move forward to the first caregiving stage after Pre-Alzheimer's disease: the Early-to-Mild Stage.

About YOU

Now is the time to concentrate on you. Make a chart about yourself answering the same questions aforementioned. You are in the Pre-Alzheimer's stage—living with your own strengths and weaknesses, "likes" and "dislikes." What purposes/goals do you have for your life? What are your passions? What stimulates your mind, body, and spirit?

Compare your loved one's Pre-Alzheimer's disease chart with your own—looking at your information under Memory, Language, Complex Tasks, Social Skills, and Senses. Recognize where you match and where you don't match. Throughout your caregiving partnership in the Early-to-Mild Stage and part of the Moderate Stage, don't force yourself to do recreational things that you do not like. If your loved one likes to play cards and you don't, ask someone else to come visit for an afternoon of cards and refreshments. Use other persons on your team to substitute for you when you can.

The basic information about your loved one and yourself may be revised throughout this long process. Right now, the lists can help you to keep focused on your goals of giving dignified, appropriate, and safe care for your loved one and to keep yourself healthy—mind, body, and spirit—while finding ways to enrich your life each and every day.

Keeping yourself focused on what can be done and what can't be done is important. Look for ways to help you be enthusiastic about giving care. Try new things for both of you. Being flexible while making adjustments for your loved one and yourself throughout the caregiving process is very important.

THE EARLY-TO-MILD STAGE OF CAREGIVING: WHAT DO CAREGIVERS NEED?

Here is some "Advice from a Person with Alzheimer's Disease."

- Don't hurry me. Hurrying me tends to make me forget, and then I get confused.
- If I forget something, remind me gently. If I seem to forget that company is coming or that we are due to be somewhere, help me realize that it is okay if we are a little late or that everything needed is not ready.
- Do not ask me questions. This frustrates me and makes me feel I am being tested.
- When I forget, either laugh with me or hug me, but please do not try to make excuses for me. When you do that, it makes me angry and I feel that you do not understand what I am feeling inside.
- When I say, "I don't know how to turn on the oven," just come and help me. No words are needed, and chances are tomorrow I may be able to do it on my own.
- When I tell you something "dumb" that I did, please listen and try to understand that what I am really trying to tell you is that I am scared and hurting. I need to be loved and given time to talk about what is happening to me.
- When I am silent and unable to sleep, chances are I am struggling with my own fears about how this is going to hurt you as time goes on. I am asking myself what is going to happen to me and how we as a family are going to cope and survive.

- Try to understand that some days I almost convince myself there is nothing wrong with me... and then there are days when I have no doubt that my head is not working normally. These latter days are the ones when you're most apt to find me down in spirit.
- Try to understand that I am finding it difficult to believe that this is really happening to me. The big questions, "why?" and "how long?" keep going on in my head.

[By Jeanne Capp, an early stage Alzheimer's patient. Member of the Early Stage Alzheimer's Support Group of Marlborough, New Hampshire.]

During this stage of the disease—using their own powers of reflection— many persons with dementia know there is something wrong with their abilities to do the things they used to do. They tell us they are worried when they find themselves getting lost when traveling to familiar places. They tell us they realize that learning new ways to do things at work is more difficult and sometimes too difficult to perform. They know they are not recognizing persons' faces, names, and so on, as they used to. They know they can still do many things, but they are worried about the changes they perceive. There is confusion about when your loved one needs help and when your loved one can perform tasks on his/her own. Sometimes they say: "Why do I need help? Why am I doing things I don't intend to do? My world is changing, and I can't control it! I am anxious about many things...."

You have probably heard stories about persons who have Alzheimer's disease. You have heard about what "can" happen in a worst case scenario. But the things you have read may not necessarily happen in your caregiving situation. In my years of caregiving, I read many things that scared me because I did not have the insight to say to myself:

- All these things COULD happen, but I am caring for only THIS person at this time.
- I need to concentrate on what IS happening, not what MAY happen in the future.
- I need to become more disciplined and live in the present moment.

It is much easier to concentrate on what is happening in the present rather than worrying yourself about what might happen in the future. Maybe that is why the Lord's Prayer says: "Give us this day our daily bread."

Using this chart, review the shaded area and notice that the main change in your loved one's abilities involves memory (Figure 7.2). But that change can affect much of your loved one's life and your life.

About Your Loved One

In this Early-to-Mild Stage, your loved one can function independently for some period of time. If your loved one is diagnosed with Alzheimer's disease, then more of your time is going to be needed to give care to him/her. This is the time for you to consider the demands on your life and the resources you have to call upon. At the beginning of this stage of 3 to 5 years in length, your loved one can continue to drive for a time, be employed, and participate in family and community activities.

About You

You know as a caregiver that things are changing for you, too. Your role as a caregiver now is to offer support, encouragement, and companionship. You are finding that you need to give more assistance with some daily activities and planning for the future. If you were giving care for other physical ailments before the diagnosis of Alzheimer's disease or a related dementia and that took about 10 percent of your time, now you will move to caregiving for 15 to 20 percent of your time. It is time to assess your life style and make modifications where it is most needed.

There is no one recipe that fits all. That is why this book is titled, *The Alzheimer's Caregiving Puzzle: Putting Together the Pieces*. We can lead you to your own personal answers about how to take care of yourself at this stage of the disease.

Understand Yourself as a Caregiver

Evaluate your personal strengths and weaknesses as a caregiver. What am I doing well? How do I feel physically? What do I need help with? Caregiving should be a team effort. Stay connected to

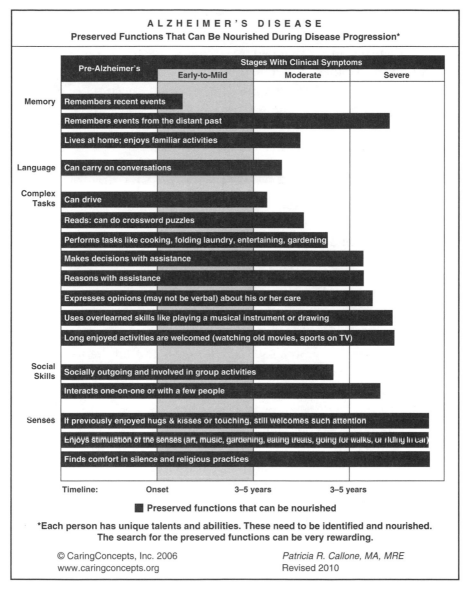

Figure 7.2   A Caregiver's Perspectives, Early-to-Mild Stage.

your life resources. Your needs will change. What assistance do you need now? What can you no longer do? What modifications do you need to make so that you can give more time to your loved one and still give yourself time to be with your family, be employed, keep up your social contacts, and so on? Who can you call to ask for assistance—family members, friends of your loved one, your own friends, your faith community's resources, and so on? Call the local chapter of the Alzheimer's Association and ask for an appointment to find their resources that can assist you.

Learn to balance the demands of your life with your caregiving duties. Are your children growing older and need more of your time? Is your husband able to flex his time at work and help you more? Can you flex your time at work? Are there neighbors who can sit with your loved one while you do other things?

Monitor your attitude about caregiving. How is your energy holding up? Are you beginning to resent the extra time it takes to care for your loved one? Are you "taking quiet time" for yourself? Are you consciously trying to find humor in the little things that seem to interrupt daily life? Be mindful of the ways in which you are growing as a caregiver. What are you learning about yourself as you continue your caregiving duties? Are you learning to balance life more than you did before? Give yourself credit for the good you are doing and learn from your mistakes.

Keep communication open all the time. Be aware of transitions during the caregiving process. Look for clues to find the right piece of the puzzle to put together to make the picture you want: giving dignified, appropriate, and safe care to your loved one and to enrich your life (mind, body, and spirit) throughout the caregiving process. Make certain you keep all medical appointments for yourself.

The "Meet My Loved One" booklet you are putting together will be a constant tool that can be used throughout all of the stages of the caregiving process. You can add to the booklet now. Record for yourself and your family the changes that are taking place. The booklet should become a valuable tool for everyone on your team.

This is the time to use the "Memory Prompts" in your booklet. The memory prompts cover the years 1920 to 2009. They are taken in part from *Remember When … A Nostalgic Look Back in Time* and have been added to by many people who have lived through those years. Some of the information helps give your loved one a picture of a time in history through which he/she lived. Your loved one may like reminiscing when a loaf of bread cost 20¢, a bottle of milk cost 1.04¢, a gallon of gas cost 25¢, and so on.

Notice, we are concentrating on the pleasant memories that you want to relive together—not the unpleasant things that have happened in life. (Your loved one may forget that someone has died. If your loved one asks, "How is Uncle Hank?" and you know that he has died, just answer, "Fine." Don't remind your loved one that Uncle Hank has died because then the whole process of grieving may take place again.) When you concentrate on pleasant memories with your loved one, it gives the person a sense of reliving the pleasant past. Continue to be nurturing in all the functions your loved one can still use. Continue to call on your caregiving team members for help.

You can offer support, encouragement, companionship, and create an environment that becomes more of a routine and familiar to your loved one. You want to maintain an environment that is predictable for both of you. Most of the time, caregivers are not certain of when to let the person with Alzheimer's disease be in control and when not to. Transitioning from the Early-to-Mild Stage to the Moderate Stage of the disease is very difficult. Look for the clues and cues your loved one gives you and make changes that are needed.

THE MODERATE STAGE OF CAREGIVING: WHAT DO CAREGIVERS NEED?

About Your Loved One

This is the time when persons with dementia notice that their losses are becoming more apparent and permanent; that they are having trouble driving and the family does not want them to drive; that more is going on with their minds; and that they cannot keep up with their familiar, daily living activities. They are now living with the losses experienced in the Early-to-Mild Stage of the disease (mostly memory) and are beginning to experience the losses that appear during the Moderate Stage.

Review the shaded part of the chart to help you realize the many changes that may be taking place because Alzheimer's disease is progressing across the brain (Figure 7.3). Try to understand that you can't stop the changes from taking place. But you can find ways to handle the changes that are appropriate for you and your loved one.

As you review the chart, you can see the functions that are becoming less available to the person with Alzheimer's disease

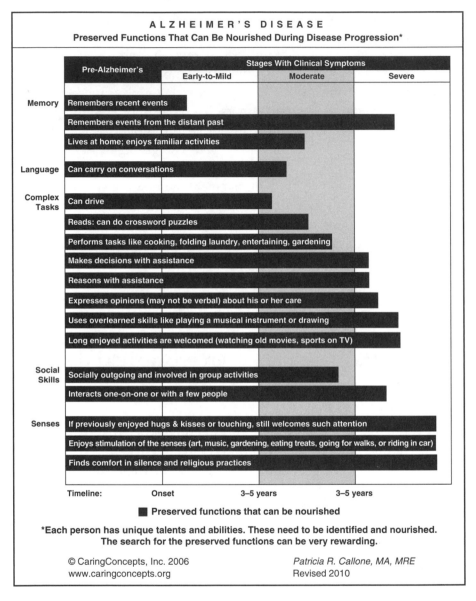

Figure 7.3   A Caregiver's Perspective, Moderate Stage.

or related dementia. In addition, there is more decline in his/her memory. The Moderate Stage of caregiving appears to be the longest caregiving stage and more difficult for caregivers. Your loved one's behavior may change. He/she may become more irritable, begin to become more apathetic, may have trouble with sleeping through the night, and may begin to wander. Your loved one may have difficulty in expressing his/her thoughts, have more trouble getting dressed, may jumble words when trying to carry on a conversation, and may rely on gestures to communicate rather than words. During this caregiving stage your loved one will probably lose the ability to drive and thus become more dependent on you and others.

Driving is one of the hardest issues to handle. You and others may notice that your loved one cannot drive safely any more. But your loved one does not want to give up driving—until something happens that shows himself/herself and everyone else that driving the car is no longer an activity that your loved one should do.

Of course persons become frightened because of these changes. Of course sometimes they withdraw from conversations because they can't keep up. Of course they don't want to lose their licenses and become dependent on others. Of course there are changes in the way they act because they are afraid and anxious about how they will continue to live their own lives. Of course they fight to be independent. The losses continue and sometimes become a surprise to your loved one and you. Here is where you, as caregiver, need to find ways to tell your loved one that he/she is safe and loved.

About You

Here is where more of your time that was spent on something else—family, friends, and work—can tend to be cut because of more responsibilities you are now being asked to handle. This is the "danger time" for you as primary caregiver. Here is where you need to talk with others (friends, family, and faith leaders) to get some perspective on your own life and health. Here is where most of the emotional stress of caregiving takes place. Here is where your own health can begin to suffer; your own family relationships suffer; and your duties and responsibilities at work suffer. Here is where you can become more irritable—because you are also frightened about what is taking place.

What would you tell a friend if he/she were in your position? Now is a time for you to make adjustments for your own spiritual, physical, emotional, intellectual, and social health. Take your own advice and review the following:

Keep Focused on Your Two Goals

- To give dignified, appropriate, and safe care to your loved one throughout the progression of the disease
- To enrich your own life in mind, body, and spirit

Understand Yourself as Caregiver, as Your Needs May Change.

Your loved one is changing, and your life is changing, too. Evaluate your personal strengths and weaknesses now. If you were spending about 20 to 25 percent of your time caregiving in the Early-to-Mild Stage of the disease, more time will be needed for caregiving in the Moderate Stage. You may now feel as if you should be giving from 30 to 40 percent of your time to your loved one.

Once again, this really should be a team effort. Stay connected to your life resources. You may not be able to give more time to caregiving because of your own physical, mental, and spiritual capacities. It is time once again to call on your team of resources and ask for help in the particular situation's like helping with bathing or dressing. What resources/help do you need now?

Learn to balance the demands of your life and caregiving duties. Other family members (brothers and sisters) may not have contributed to giving care to your loved one before this time. Now is their time to support you and help you get or keep balance in your life. To other family members (your spouse and children), the person with Alzheimer's disease seems to be taking all the energy and love you have to give. Your family may be missing your presence with them. Families understand for awhile, but can become impatient with the caregiver as the months of caregiving continue. Sometimes you, as primary caregiver, need to say, "I cannot continue to do these things any more: (Name them). I can continue to do these things: (Name them). Someone else needs to do these things: (Name them).

Find and use resources in your community or have someone help you find the resources you need like: Meals on Wheels from your state's area Office on Aging to help with food; use volunteers from church or hired help from agencies who do non-medical in-home care. Use the resources of your faith community to visit with your loved one. Call on all the medical and agency resources that are available. Use online resources—especially those provided by the National Alzheimer's association: www.alz.org.

Be mindful of the ways in which you are growing as a caregiver. Have you found yourself becoming more compassionate in living with the changes in others' lives and yours? Are you sharing some of the ways you are giving care with other caregivers in families you know? Have you become more reflective about your own life as well as the lives of other loved ones in your family? Are your perspectives changing about what is really important in life and what is not? Are you finding that you are more self-disciplined in caregiving to your loved one in that you can "wait" for the person to do what he/she can do and praise him/her for taking care of the responsibilities that he/she can handle?

Here are some challenges for living with your loved one. In this stage of caregiving, you want to be able to find ways:

- To stimulate your loved one in the areas he/she likes and you like—because this will give you pleasure too
- To socialize with your loved one in areas he/she likes and you like—because this will give you pleasure too
- To keep your loved one safe—and yourself safe. Perhaps your loved one's body is getting too heavy to lift. Get help. Don't strain your body in trying to help
- To find a daily rhythm that fits both of your lives—that you enjoy—because this will give you pleasure too
- To continue to look for resources from your caregiving team members

Continue to add to the "Meet My Loved One" booklet that you started. What projects or activities can still be done? What can't? What is enjoyable? What is humorous about life at this time? Revise the lists and charts so that other family members can see changes that are occurring. Look at the charts you made about yourself. Are your "likes and dislikes" changing? Recognize what you can do and what you cannot do. Be aware of the transitions that are taking place.

Keep Communication Open All the Time

During the end of the Moderate Stage of caregiving, there can be more family disagreements. How long can you continue to care for your loved one? How long is he/she safe in the environment in which he/she is living? What other physical ailments are occurring for your loved one? For you? Be aware of the clues and cues your loved one is giving you at this time. This is the way he/she is communicating with you—not verbally, but with gestures, silence, smiles, and laughter. You know what all these clues and cues mean now.

There may be many transitions from the middle of the Moderate Stage to the beginning of the Severe Stage. One of my friends recently said: "Why can't we see these bodily failings as a natural process? The body has served and served and served. Why are we surprised? I wish I could just relax and see all of this as a progression of Alzheimer's disease that affects the whole body." How right she is. All of the transitions are a process of the disease progression. We, as caregivers, just need to relax and understand that not much is in our control as we continue to give care into the Severe Stage.

SEVERE STAGE OF CAREGIVING: WHAT DO CAREGIVERS NEED?

About Your Loved One

As your loved one moves from the end of the Moderate Stage to the Severe Stage, he or she may experience difficulty in eating and swallowing. Your loved one may need assistance in walking, become bedridden, or chair-bound. Your loved one may become more vulnerable to infections. Your loved one may lose the ability to communicate. Your loved one—who always loved to eat—may decide that he/she doesn't want to eat and doesn't want to live according to routines that have been established earlier. Look for the clues and cues from your loved one. He/she is still communicating what he/she wants and doesn't want. No matter what the behavior, understand that the changes are happening because of Alzheimer's disease and are not intentional.

Your loved one is still with you. He/she has grown accustomed to your loving care. The loving touch from family, friends, and other caregivers is sometimes the best way to communicate with him/her.

The progression of Alzheimer's disease across the brain is almost complete.

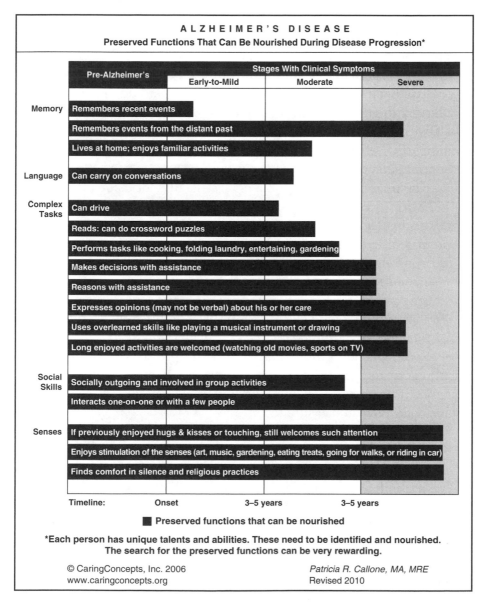

Figure 7.4   A Caregiver's Perspectives, Severe Stage.

Review the shaded part of the chart (Figure 7.4). You can see that some functions still remain. The long-remembered events can still be pleasurable for your loved one. Those events—that might be recorded in the booklet "Meet My Loved One"—can now be used to give pleasure to your loved one, yourself, and others.

About You

Many families find that they need to rely on others to do much of the personal caregiving responsibilities in the Severe Stage. If you and your family have decided to care for your loved one at home, then you will need to rely on all the resources available to you. You will need help with the care of the whole body, as well as the appropriate stimulation and rest for your loved one. Many times there are compounding complications at this stage of the disease. You may need to use hospice resources at home or go to a hospice facility for complete care.

Review the "Meet My Loved One" project that you began at the very beginning of your "caregiving partnership" with your loved one. You may have many pages of stories about your loved one's pleasant experiences, many pictures of important times that involved your loved one and his/her family.

You may have collected songs, records, and favorite stories that now mean a lot more to you and your loved family now. If your loved one wants to (or can) talk, this is the time for you to go back in your loved one's memory and stimulate his/her precious moments. You can read or talk about the stories you have collected. Your loved one can experience again the pleasurable moments you have collected. This will give you pleasure too.

Stimulate the senses with tastes and smells your loved one continues to like and you like. Play soothing music that your loved one has enjoyed. Touch your loved one with hand creams or other scents that relax you and your loved one. All of this kind of loving, personal care will give pleasure to your loved one and comfort you in these difficult days.

Your loved one may not recognize you because of the disease progression. Your loved one may have said mean things to you, but that happened because of the disease progression across the brain. You may have said mean things to your loved one. But all those things are past... and should be forgotten. So much of the "caregiving partnership" involves love and forgiveness, which you have expressed again and again. Your loved one may now spend more time sleeping, but he/she is still there.

Now is the time to review your loved one's End-of-Life Directives/Wishes. This is the time to honor them. Be peaceful as you end your caregiving partnership with your loved one who has Alzheimer's disease or related dementia. Be assured you have done a good job—the best possible caregiving for your loved one and yourself.

Cherish the "Meet My Loved One" booklet you compiled or any other memories you have of your loved one. Keep them for your family and grandchildren. They will see the courage, sacrifice, and pleasure you had when you gave care to your loved one. You will have taught them honestly and well.

CHAPTER 8

Caregiving Styles

Barbara Vasiloff

YOU: A CAREGIVER

If you are a caregiver of a person with Alzheimer's disease or other dementia, there is a good possibility that you have not received previous training for this role. You might be a grandchild, single parent, spouse, brother, sister, daughter, son, cousin, friend, or neighbor. Your caregiving role most likely began when the person for whom you are providing care showed signs that he/she was not able to perform in life as he/she used to or received the diagnosis of Alzheimer's disease.

You might have embraced this new role with joy and enthusiasm. You might believe you can help the person live with dignity and feel a sense of purpose. On the other hand, you might feel apprehensive about being a caregiver. You can be filled with self-doubt and worry during the process of caregiving. This wide range of feelings is natural and experienced by everyone at one time or another.

Alzheimer's disease will involuntarily change a person's behavior. So, even if you are an enthusiastic caregiver, you can feel helpless as you try to understand behaviors in a rational way. Conflict and tension can be experienced among family members who have different ideas about what would be the best course of action. Caregivers are challenged daily to keep the lines of communication open with their loved ones who have the disease, as well as with concerned family members and friends.

Caregivers can become enablers and take on roles the person for whom they are caring could still perform by himself/herself. One thing is certain, since Alzheimer's disease affects each person differently, caregiving is almost always on-the-job training and often trial and error. I believe the challenges you will face need not be overwhelming if you are willing to take a journey with the person for whom you are caring and make changes in your own life as the person with dementia changes.

CAREGIVERS GO THROUGH TRANSITIONS AND STAGES IN CAREGIVING

As persons with Alzheimer's disease transition through the Early-to-Mild, Moderate, and Severe Stage, so will you. This chapter is written to help you take some of the guess work out of understanding your role as a caregiver during the different stages of the disease. In this chapter, you will be introduced to three caregiving styles. Each style can help you nurture the person with Alzheimer's disease and retain your own dignity and the dignity of the one being cared for as these transitions take place. Each style indicates the amount of "power" or "control" that is given to persons with dementia and the amount of "power" or "control" you retain as their caregiver.

The styles include:

- Non-Interventionist Style, in which the person with Alzheimer's disease takes full control of life and you act as a resource person to assist him/her as needed. This has been referred to as the "YOU" Style because power is out of your hands and in the hands of the person for whom you are taking care.
- Interactionalist Style, in which you let persons for whom you are caring be in control of situations as long as they are not making decisions that can cause danger to themselves or others, are disturbing to others, or are irrational. When these situations occur you collaborate with others (persons with dementia as well as other family members) and make shared decisions. Because consultation with others is needed at this point in caregiving, this style has been referred to as the "WE" Style of caregiving.
- Interventionist Style, in which you take the lead on almost all of the daily decisions that need to be made. The more you know about the wishes of the persons for whom you

are caring, the better you will be able to make decisions that will be in their best interest. Because you retain almost all of the control, this style has been referred to as the "I" Style of caregiving.

As you read the descriptions of the three styles of caregiving, perhaps situations will pop into your head of times when you have worked out of each of the styles. These different ways of giving care can be used many times during one day, but your preferred style will become prominent when you:

- Are involved in a conflict
- Are tired or haven't been taking care of yourself
- Are involved in a new situation that hasn't occurred before
- Have little time to think about what would be best for you and the person for whom you are caring; and most importantly
- During the different stages of the disease

Your *preferred* style may not be the one that best nurtures the person with dementia. If you understand these styles, you can switch a style when the one you prefer is no longer nurturing. As I reflected on the caregiving I have provided in the past 4 years, I recognize that as my mom transitioned through the Early-to-Mild, Moderate, and Severe stages of dementia each of the three caregiving styles became more prominent in my life. As you read about each stage, you will note how I, as the caregiver, transitioned along with my mom.

My hope is that you will see this as a mutual journey made by people who believe a loving relationship can transcend any difficult situation into an opportunity to show care.

THE FIRST TRANSITION: THE "YOU" STYLE OF CAREGIVING

My full-time caregiving began three-and-half years ago when I moved from Omaha, Nebraska, where I had lived for 35 years to Reedsville, Pennsylvania, a small town nestled in the mountains of central Pennsylvania. At that time Dad, who was 92 years old, had suffered a mini-stroke which left him with few, if any, noticeable side effects.

Mom, who was 91, had been taking Aricept for years to help with short-term memory loss, as she tended to repeat questions and comments frequently. They lived in their own home, and I lived with them while I searched for a place of my own. I rented an office for my business and spent time looking at properties. When time permitted, we were able to take overnight trips to NY and Maryland and other parts of Pennsylvania to visit relatives and vacation.

Going to church, eating out, and playing cards every Sunday were three social events the folks looked forward to. Mom read the newspaper every day and several different magazines. Dad cut the grass, took out the garbage, and did most of the outside chores. He paid all the bills, opened mail, and asked me to help him balance the checkbook each month because his macular degeneration made it difficult for him to see. He did monitor his blood sugar reading each day and insisted on taking his own pills rather than let me dispense them as I did with Mom, since she would forget to take them. Mom cleaned, cooked, washed clothes, did dishes, and visited with neighbors. At this point, they were both highly functional.

I didn't worry about going to the office for 4 or 5 hours and leaving them at home, or giving two day workshops out of the city. A phone call to check in on them was enough to let me know they were safe and doing well.

One of the first things Dad wanted to do when I moved back was to visit his lawyer and update his will. During this process, he turned over his durable power of attorney to me, and both he and Mom signed Living Wills. We had a funeral director visit the home, and arrangements for both Mom and Dad were made and paid for. I helped Dad organize a three-ring binder into which he put all his CDs, investments, insurance policies, bank statements, etc. In another, we put birth certificates, marriage license, passport, power of attorney papers, the will, funeral arrangements, and receipts for paid cemetery plots.

It was evident to me that Dad had been compensating for Mom's loss of memory in several ways. He answered the phone so he could tell her who was on the phone before she got on. He invented the acronym CEO which stood for cereal, eggs, oatmeal and used it to help her remember what to fix for breakfast. I noticed he was often short tempered with her because she was hard of hearing and he didn't like repeating things. I quickly fell into the same pattern. While my folks were definitely in control of their lives, I was there to assist as needed, when asked, or to suggest things that would make life easier for them. One of the first things I did was have Mom's hearing tested. She was fit for hearing aids because of nerve damage in each ear; wearing them made life better for all of us.

My caregiving style at this point can be defined as a Non-Interventionist. This is a technical term that simply means, as a caregiver, I allowed the power or control to rest with my folks. I acted as an advocate and resource and nurtured them by allowing them to be as independent as possible. As caregiver, I had a life independent from theirs, and our lives were mutually enhanced by one another.

Because they retained control over their decisions and desires and I did not intervene, this style has been referred to as the "YOU" Style of caregiving. Had I tried to take over control of situations or suggested they do things differently than their routine, my help would not have been so welcomed. Being new to caregiving, using this style suited me well as I have always been extremely independent and enjoyed being with others who had this same trait.

FURTHER EXPLANATION OF THE "YOU" CAREGIVING STYLE

- The "YOU" Style tends to work best during the Early-to-Mild stage of a person's dementia, when he or she can still make judgments and is aware of what is happening—even during times of forgetfulness.
- The "YOU" Style allows caregivers to give their loved ones power to have control over their own lives.
- The "YOU" Style lets caregivers yield to the needs of loved ones and give persons the dignity of their own choices.

- The "YOU" Style is healthy for all concerned, as long as persons with dementia are safe and caregivers understand changes are occurring.
- The "YOU" Style is the only style caregivers can have in the early stages of Alzheimer's if loved ones are strong willed and will not listen to others.

When you use the "YOU" Style of caregiving you:

- Act as an advocate and resource person—You ask persons with dementia what they need or want.
- Encourage others—Compliment persons with dementia for trying to accomplish tasks even if they are not perfect when done.
- Focus on positive qualities—Look at the person's actions and point out what is good.
- Are an active listener—You don't solve problems; you just repeat back what the person has told you, showing you understand.
- Communicate effectively—Speak simply and check for understanding.
- Are sensitive to the feelings of others—Notice the emotions of persons and ask if they are having a good day or bad day.
- Ask for what you need—You tell persons when you can or cannot be there for them.
- Remain comfortable while discussing sensitive subjects— Talk about end of life issues and help them make necessary arrangements.
- Can observe without interfering—Are present with persons and sometimes sit with them in silence.
- Are viewed as accessible by others—You tell persons when and how to reach you and help them feel comfortable discussing their needs or concerns.

In the Early-to-Mild Stage, you can feel comfortable using the "YOU or Non-Interventionist Style if you can answer "Yes" to most of these questions:

- Is the person capable of living independently?

- Will the person be safe in spite of his/her forgetfulness?
- Does the person want to be helpful and can he/she follow instructions?
- Is the person able to make sound judgments?
- Is the person generally aware during times of forgetfulness?
- Is the person strong-willed and unable to take directions from others?
- Has the person told you that he/she is not ready for someone to take care of his/her needs?
- Are you able to let go of your opinions and ideas and follow the lead from persons who have dementia?

THE SECOND TRANSITION: THE "WE" STYLE OF CAREGIVING

There came a point when I could no longer answer "Yes" to most of these questions. I found myself still living in my folk's home a year and a half later. It became evident that buying a home would only mean I would never live in it. Mom gave many clues that she needed more assistance. She began to burn the food on the stove. She would put something on the stove and then walk away or forget it was cooking. She allowed me to take the lead on meals and would ask to assist by making salads or cleaning vegetables, but not using the stove or oven. When it came time to do the shopping, she would say, "You go. You can get it done faster without me." Or "I really don't want to go. Do I have to?"

One day, I opened the cabinet under the bathroom sink and was shocked to find 20 pairs of soiled underwear. When changing, Mom would place them there thinking she would hand wash them as she once did, but now she forgot they were there. She asked to have the blind on the porch lowered so neighbors wouldn't see her when she wanted to go out to sit.

Every four months when her doctor would administer the Cognitive Functioning Quiz, she would lose several more points. The doctor started her on Naminda in addition to the Aricept. He called her condition senile dementia. Tests showed no blockage in the arteries leading to the brain.

Dad's sight now prevented him from driving, and he gave up his keys and his car. I helped him with the mowing by doing the front lawn while he did the back. He couldn't comprehend that Mom was not intentionally doing some of the things she did and became very impatient with her. Every time we were out, I would coach him, "Dad, Mom isn't doing these things on purpose. She really can't remember. It is a disease in her brain. It doesn't help when you get mad at her." What made him most angry was her constant hiding of money. If he left a check on his dresser, he would find it missing. Mom would have placed it in his top drawer for him so the imaginary "someone's" wouldn't take it. She hid money everywhere. Finally, in desperation, he collected all of it and put it in one pouch. He called it "their pot." He told her anytime she wanted money, all she had to do was ask, and he would give her more than she asked for.

As the caregiver, I often acted as a mediator. I interpreted for Mom what Dad was saying and interpreted for Dad what Mom was doing. My sisters and brother, who all lived in other states, began to feel a sense of guilt that they were not able to help more. I gave them a schedule of weeks when I would need one of them to take over for me. They were all generous with their time and arranged to be here during the times I needed to be away. I cut back on my work load and sent others to give workshops that I would normally have given. I found myself taking on more of the household duties... cooking, laundry, cleaning, and the one job that was the toughest for me, being their social director.

I began to look forward to Sunday afternoons when I could drop the folks off with one of Dad's sisters to play cards for several hours. It was the only time I felt free from the responsibility of being the primary caregiver. I needed Dad's sisters to help when I called them. As long as I let go of my personal agendas and stayed present to the needs of the moment, I was able to lovingly care for the folks. When my agenda came first, there was a constant tension between feeling like a failure in the caregiving process and feeling like I needed to do things for myself for self-preservation. As a transition took place in the health of my folks, it necessitated a transition in me. I took on more roles, and I moved from using the Non-Interventionist or

'YOU" Style of caregiving to an Interactionalist or "WE" Style. I capitalized on the activities Mom and Dad still demonstrated a capacity for and supplemented those they were no longer able to do. We shared control over the household and I was forced to face my limitations and enlist the help of others as needed.

FURTHER EXPLANATION OF THE "WE" CAREGIVING STYLE

In the Moderate Stage of dementia, persons with dementia show signs (give "Clues") of not being able to care for themselves as much as in the Early-to-Mild Stage of the disease and need help and direction from caregivers for their own safety.

During the Moderate Stage of dementia, the Interactionalist or "WE" Style tends to work best when caregivers have been educated to know what works best as changes take place in the brain. In the "We" Style, family members are involved as much as possible in understanding the disease and seeking solutions to future questions. Families can schedule regular times to meet to discuss progress and assign different family members the task of finding resources and programs for support or knowledge about the disease and what to do next.

In the "WE" Style, caregivers let persons with dementia be as self-sufficient as possible, but still hold the power in the relationship to make decisions for their safety and well-being. When you use the "WE" Style of caregiving you:

- Act as a negotiator—Interpret actions and meanings to other family members who might not see the total needs of the one for whom you are caring.
- Understand the need for socialization for the loved one and yourself—Involve other people in their lives and make time for rest and relaxation for yourself.
- Share time, talents, and treasures as best you can—Take one day at a time and know you will not do everything perfectly but will do all with love and genuine concern.
- Expect different viewpoints and opinions—Know that there will always be three viewpoints: The "YOU" point of view; the

"WE" point of view; and the "I" point of view. Think about what will best meet the needs of the person for whom you are caring.

- Expect to take the lead sometimes and give the lead over at times—Be an advocate for persons with the disease and carry out their wishes as best you can.
- Understand the rights and responsibilities of all involved—Take the lead when your loved one demonstrates actions that are dangerous, disruptive, or illogical.
- Rely on outside resources and experts—Review catalogues that contain independent living devices and purchase those that will be helpful.
- Be comfortable in delegating tasks—Turn care over to others so you can have respite as needed.

In the Moderate Stage, you can feel comfortable using the "WE" Style if you can answer "Yes" to most of these questions:

- Has a diagnosis of Alzheimer's disease been made by a physician with expertise in dementia?
- Are you becoming less able to meet the basic needs of the person for whom you are caring?
- Do you find yourself becoming overwhelmed or depressed or worried a majority of the time?
- Are family members and friends showing concerns and asking to be part of the long-term care process?
- Are you concerned about the safety needs of the person in your care?
- Has the person with dementia indicated that he/she would like to go places or do things, but cannot do so independently?
- Is there conflict among family members regarding the methods of care the person with dementia should receive?

You may be able to answer "Yes" to these questions early on in the progression of the disease, but usually in the Moderate Stage, the need to share the decision-making power becomes apparent. The task of balancing caregiving for others and your needs will begin to come into conflict. It will become necessary to delegate some of the caregiving to other professionals, friends, and family members using the "team" of caregiving. Allow yourself to do this. At this stage, you can no longer let loved ones have full power over their lives, but you cannot assume full control either.

THE THIRD TRANSITION: THE "I" STYLE OF CAREGIVING

I have now remodeled the basement and moved my office into my folks' home so I can be available 24/7. I disposed of more personal furnishings to make room for the three of us to live together.

Mom's ability to reason and make independent judgments has gradually diminished over the past three years. She will frequently ask, "What can I do now?" or say, "You decide. You know best." Mom now waits for directions from me to tell her how and when to dress, bathe, eat, sit on the porch, rest, etc. The embarrassment she initially had when I would help her undress and get into the bathtub is gone. Her willingness to help outweighs her ability to perform even simple tasks. She questions whether two placemats, three, or more should be set out for the three of us each day. She can't decide if she should put out tablespoons or teaspoons. And if asked to stir something in a pan, she will do so for three or four times and then wander off leaving things to burn. I have learned to solicit her help as often as possible, giving her tasks I know she can still perform. Her desire to be productive is so evident I am compelled to search for things she can do. When she asks, "What is there for me to do?" I feel quite sure she is asking about her limitations as well as productive work.

One of the things she does with eagerness is shred unwanted or important papers. I purchased a heavy duty shredder from Sam's Club and gathered papers that needed to be shred. Just as my supply was running out, two visitors from church came to the house. As we visited, they noticed the large shredder and asked about it. When the church moved its office from one location to another, they uncovered boxes of forms dating back 20 years. "If you are serious about helping us out, we will gladly bring you materials to shred," they said. For weeks afterwards, boxes and boxes of papers were delivered to our house. This started a process that continues today, not just for one church but for three. Each morning after breakfast, Mom and Dad will do about an hour of shredding. It is their job, and they like helping the church. Mom takes her other job of caring for Dad just as seriously. If she leaves the room where he is sitting, she will immediately ask, "Where's Dad?" forgetting from moment to moment.

Dad had a major stroke 15 months ago. He spent 12 weeks in rehab and a nursing home. His right arm and hand still has paralysis, and his long- and short-term memory has also diminished. He was released from the home with me guaranteeing that I would now be his caregiver 24/7. Home health nurses and physical therapists came for about 8 weeks, but when he showed no signs of further decline, Medicare no longer would fund his care. Had Dad welcomed these helpers into his home, private pay was and is always an option. But Dad was eager for them to be finished with their therapy and stop coming into the sanctity of his home. When he needs help with bathing and personal care, enlisting the help of the Hospice Palliative Care unit will be one decision I will make despite his protests.

While in rehab Dad was given a small dose of insulin each day. As a caregiver, one of the most difficult adjustments I had to make was to give Dad this daily insulin shot. I tried but was unable to find a nurse who could come at a prescribed time each day. I woke with a sick stomach and a cold sweat each morning until the shot was finally given. Other caregivers told me to "Toughen it out. You'll get used to it." But I never did. Within a few weeks at my urging, his primary doctor took him off the insulin and substituted another pill, which has worked well to control his diabetes.

My time is measured by the pills that have to be dispersed throughout the day—11 different pills for Dad and 5 different ones for Mom. Some pills have to be given 15 minutes before meals, others with meals, and still others at 11 a.m. and before bed time. Card playing continues. We now play with a deck of cards that are 7 inches by 4 inches with only 7 cards to make sets or runs. Both Mom and Dad still enjoy playing, but they can play for 3 to 4 hours at a time, and I simply cannot do this. I arranged to have one of their friends, who is 81, to come every Friday afternoon to play from 2 p.m. to 5:00 p.m. and another volunteer from our church comes on Wed. from 2 p.m. to 4 p.m. When the family visits and asks what they can do to help, I always say, "Play cards with them, and just sit with them." Sometimes I think I will never enjoy a good card game again when this caregiving is over.

Another tough adjustment for me is their total lack of communication. I read to them from the daily newspaper, but they make no comments about the stories read. Mom will gesture when she wants me to pour milk or pass something on the table. She will say one word and expect me to know what she is trying to communicate. When asked to make a choice such as what foods sound good for dinner, she will say, "I'm not hungry." At her last doctor's appointment, she lost 5 pounds.

Last September, Mom and Dad celebrated their 70th wedding anniversary, and our family gathered for a quiet celebration. During this time, we remembered the larger parties that took place on their 50th and 60th anniversaries, looking at videos and picture albums that were made at the time. We certainly made the right decision keeping the celebration small. They received over 50 cards, had several Catholic masses said for them, and on Sunday we just had cake and fruit and invited Dad's three sisters over to help celebrate. After dinner, my brother tried to tell Mom and Dad how much we were grateful for the gift they gave us of being married for 70 years. He spoke sensitively from his heart for several minutes trying to make himself clearly understood. When he stopped, Dad, who had been listening intently said, "What was the gift?" My brother said it reminded him of the time he was seriously explaining to his son Alex, who was then 6 or 7, how to hold a baseball bat and then swing. Alex listened intently—or so George thought— and when George was finished and asked if he understood, all Alex said was, "Dad, did you use deodorant this morning?"

Humor can easily be found in life's situations when you are a caregiver, and what a relief it is!

My folks are separating from this world, and I feel blessed to be part of this process. At the same time, watching the process is emotionally taxing because I am apprehensive about what their final moments might be like. To stay balanced, I begin my day with a short spiritual reading that has one good thought that I live with throughout the day. I force myself to walk on the treadmill each day for a minimum of 20 minutes and usually feel better when this is done. I correspond with friends on e-mail and complete personal work around their schedule. They have been sleeping until 10 a.m. or 10:30 a.m. and going to bed by 9:30 p.m. or 10 p.m., so I safeguard that time to relax and refresh myself. I make all the decisions now and try to do things the way I know they liked them to be done in the past. Since I retain most of the control, this style can be termed an Interventionist Style or "I" Style. My focus is meeting their basic needs for food, shelter, clean clothing and hygiene, and a pleasant environment in their own home. I know two things for certain. Mom and Dad want to be together for as long as possible, and they want to stay in their own home.

FURTHER EXPLANATION OF THE "I" CAREGIVING STYLE

In the Severe Stage, persons with dementia cannot take care of themselves, and as their caregiver, you will see "Clues" that tell you to take control and execute the desires of persons with dementia as they stated earlier in their lives. You will generally not be able to care for loved ones without substantial assistance near the end of life.

- The "I" Style tends to work best during the later or severe stage of persons with dementia, when they are no longer able to make decisions.
- In the "I" Style, caregivers act upon the desires of loved ones, which were discussed prior to this stage.

- In the "I" Style, caregivers have the power to make end-of-life decisions for persons with Alzheimer's disease or related dementia.
- The "I" Style works best if loved ones are in danger, are abusive, exhibit out-of-control behaviors, or are incapable of making rational decisions.
- The "I" Style works best when time, resources, or personnel to give care have become depleted.

When you use the "I" Style of caregiving you:

- Use direct, authoritative approaches—You know the person with Alzheimer's disease so well you can represent his/her needs and wishes and have signed documents that show you are his/her representative.
- Know the person you are caring for needs guidelines and limits—You know when a person is feeling fatigued or is having a bad day and protect the person from visitors or unnecessary interruptions.
- Feel comfortable taking the lead—There is a calm and peace about you that lets others know you are comfortable representing the person with dementia.
- Are highly organized and attentive to details—All prescriptions are attended to with care and medicines ordered when needed.
- Use clear judgment and rationales—Decisions are made that allow the person with dementia to keep his/her dignity. You nurture the life that remains.
- Tend to be systematic—You understand how important routines are for the person with dementia.
- Can be counted on in times of crises—You have altered your own schedule to be present for the person during his/her final days.

In this style, you take the lead and provide a plan of action. In this stage, you will keep all the power and simply make the decisions. Use this style if you can answer "Yes" to most of these questions:

- Have you been given Durable Power of Attorney—the authority to make decisions for financial matters and health care?
- Are the financial and material resources of the person with Alzheimer's disease becoming depleted?
- Is the person unable to comprehend the contents and implications of signing legal documents?
- Are you as a caregiver comfortable taking the lead and making difficult decisions?
- Is your judgment clear and have you taken into consideration the pros and cons of your actions?
- Can you be counted on to act rationally in times of stress or crisis?

There is comfort in knowing that throughout the progression of Alzheimer's disease, three interactive caregiving styles will be necessary. Understanding and using these three styles properly— giving over all control, sharing control, and taking the lead—can be invaluable as the challenges of the disease become apparent.

As a caregiver, you bring unique strengths and weaknesses to the role. People who know themselves and their own needs and are in touch with their spirituality often make the best caregivers. Compassionate caregivers learn to do their best for the person for whom they are caring one day at a time. They let the future unfold rather than anticipate the challenges that might be present in a month or year from now. They seek out others who can address areas of concern and enhance the care that is already being given. Caregiving to older persons is a "vocation" or calling in itself. Not every person is suited to do it. If you have been given the responsibility to care for older persons with Alzheimer's disease or related dementia, you can make the caregiving process a meaningful, growth process for yourself as well as for the person with dementia.

CHAPTER 9

Potential Personal Pitfalls for Caregivers

Barbara Markey and Charles Timothy Dickel

As you put together the unique Alzheimer's caregiving puzzle that is your life, there are some facts that touch the lives of all people that you will need to view through your personal lens. This chapter will look at three such realities. Any one could be a potential pitfall for you.

1. *What's the emotional system that drives how your family works?*
2. *What does Grief look like when you still have the person you are losing?*
3. *What happens if you judge yourself as guilty of "not being good enough" as a caregiver?*

The more you can name and deal with your answers to these questions, the more you will be able to care for and nurture yourself. In this book, you have been learning about Alzheimer's disease and other dementia. You have examined styles of caregiving and what you need during the stages of the disease. Now, you will spend time with some bottom-line issues that touch all of your life: family, grief, and guilt. Let your awareness of "what's going on" in you with these realities be part of your strength. They don't have to be pitfalls that get in your way.

FAMILY DYNAMICS

A family is a unit. It is not just separate people standing side-by-side. Family members are emotionally connected whether they are spread

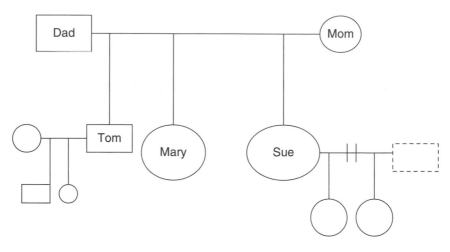

Figure 9.1   Smith family before Alzheimer's disease.

apart by many miles or living close together, whether they feel distant or have warm relationships.

Think of your family system as a *mobile*, an artwork of pieces connected by wires and sticks and hanging from the ceiling. If you change the shape and size of one piece, then the whole mobile shifts. When you add or subtract a piece, the balance of the mobile is upset and may get lopsided until the parts are arranged in a new balance (Figure 9.1).

Exercise:

1. *Draw the mobile that shows your family system before Alzheimer's disease affected it.*
2. *Draw it again as it is now.*

Exercises:

- Where am I in my family mobile? What impact has Alzheimer's had on my place and size in our family system?
- Have I noticed how Alzheimer's impacts each individual in my family? Closer? More distant? Bigger? Smaller? Changed shape or look because of anger, fear, hope, or stress?
- Ask your family members to draw their own and compare. Does it help you all to compare your perceptions?

Family members can profoundly affect each other's thoughts, feelings, and actions. You and your family members want each other's attention, approval, and support. You react to each other's expectations and distress. Even the family members from past generations or those who are dead are still part of the connectedness through remembrances of them. No two members of your family have the same shape or place in the family system. They do not have the same experience of it.

In looking at your personal situation, remember that a family system is not always created by a biological or adopted family. It may be a family born out of divorce or death and remarriage. A "family system" for you could be made up of a group of friends, colleagues, neighbors, and/or fellow church members. These may replace or add to the family you had as you were growing up. If this is the case, be aware that your original family will still have some impact on your thoughts, feelings, and actions.

> *Joe and Edna had a blended family. Both were widowed when they married and, while they loved each other, they had very different ways of dealing with problems. Joe was an engineer by training, and he attacked problems with logic and reason. Edna, on the other hand, was very emotional, and the stress of problems caused her blood pressure to soar, and she would go to pieces. Each had older children when they were married, and it was very apparent that their children's approaches to problem-solving were influenced by their respective parent. Joe's children were an actuary, two accountants, and a very structured artist; they had been heavily influenced by their father's style of problem-solving. Edna's children became very emotional in times of stress, just like their mother. When Joe became ill with dementia, there was great conflict between Joe's children and Edna and her children. They did not understand the others' ways of dealing with the challenges of Joe's illness. A major division occurred. After Joe's death, Edna cut off all communication with Joe's family.*

The "good news" is that emotional interdependence can lead families to protect, shelter, and care for their members in unity and teamwork. The "bad news" is that when one or more members get very anxious or demanding in the face of challenge or change, their feelings can become like an infection. Family connectedness can be more stressful than comforting. The "real news" is that every family system is continually changing and developing. When Alzheimer's disease strikes a family member, it strikes a family. You have an ongoing challenge to recognize what is going on in your family and to make healthy choices about how it is affecting you.

No two families are alike. Whatever the realities of your family, you can benefit from the "good news" and manage the "bad news." As you arrange and rearrange the changing puzzle before you, take time to think about four specific parts of your family puzzle.

MY FAMILY, MYSELF

I am different from my family; I am part of my family.

Members of a family are not carbon copies of each other. A healthy family system will recognize that each member is unique. Each one needs to be able to be "his or her own person." Even as individuals in a family move into their own lives, however, they are still part of the family "mobile." Family members are always connected in some degree by thoughts, feelings, and present or past actions. A family affected by Alzheimer's disease will find that not all its members think, feel, and act alike as they deal with the consequences of someone suffering from Alzheimer's. At their very best, however, the members are able to do two things: they provide both support and unity to each other; at the same time, they respect and value that each person has different views, gifts, and situations.

> *Molly is the primary caregiver for her widowed father. He has lived for several years in the home she shares with her husband and children. Now that her father has advanced Alzheimer's, she believes that she needs to find a skilled nursing home for him.*
>
> *Tom is her older brother and lives on the other side of the country. He cares deeply about his father but is seldom able to travel to see him. Instead, he tries to help by giving Molly a lot of information and suggestions long distance. She experiences*

Tom as second-guessing her decision to find more skilled care for her dad. Jane, Molly's younger sister, is a single parent with a full-time job and unable to take primary care of their father. Jane has great pain in thinking about her father in a nursing home, because "I don't think mother would have wanted us to do that." Molly feels pressured by Jane to keep their father in her home.

Molly has growing feelings of resentment for her brother and sister for not supporting her judgment. She is uncertain of herself at times. She feels as if she could lose her own good judgment because of pressure. She fears she might be losing herself and her own world because of her role as caregiver.

Families need to give both "roots" and "wings" to their members. The "roots" provide a sense of who you are and what is important to you. They give you confidence that you belong and you know that someone is always there for you. The "wings" give confidence to face new challenges or opportunities and to make decisions even in the face of conflict or criticism. You are "one with" and at the same time "uniquely you" in a healthy family system. Both your roots and your wings help you keep sight of yourself as a person who is a caregiver.

When you have a good sense of yourself, you recognize that you can also be mentally and emotionally dependent on others. At the same time, you know that you are okay as your own person. You can do and decide things yourself. This interdependence helps you stay calm and clear-headed when there is disagreement or rejection.

You can distinguish when your thinking is based on a clear assessment of the facts and not based primarily on emotion or pressure. This calm and clear sense of yourself means that you do not always have to please others. Neither do you have to routinely oppose others or bully them to conform to what you think.

After weeks of self-searching and discussion with her husband and family, Molly made her decision. She called her brother Tom and asked him to fly in for a long weekend of discussion about their father's condition. She asked Jane to arrange her job and child care, so the three of them could spend time together, be with their father, and make some decisions for his care.

Saturday morning, Molly shared with her brother and sister the struggle she was having. She told them that she heard their concerns and ideas. She still believed that her father needed to be in a nursing home. Molly talked about the needs of her own family and marriage and her inability to provide proper care at this stage of her father's illness. She asked them for help in finding a new solution for her father's care, because soon she would no longer be able to have him in her home. Both Tom and Jane were stunned. They had not realized the situation was at this point.

After the painful but honest sharing of the weekend, Molly felt better about herself. She knew that she had more understanding and support both from and for Jane and Tom. They had agreed to visit and discuss some of the care facilities she suggested. They had begun to figure out the finances. They had begun to set some timelines. They would all be involved in the next step.

It is important to balance two factors when you are dealing with the person who has Alzheimer's or with other family members and extended caregivers. Recognize that you do have need for their acceptance, approval, and support of you. Recognize also that you have need to let your thinking and your choices be guided by careful consideration of the facts and your principles. You serve no one well if you lose yourself as you depend on your background and your family support (Figure 9.2).

EMOTIONAL CONNECTIONS

Times of stress tend to show the weaknesses and strengths of any family or system. Stress is necessary to expose the limits of an individual or family's ability to adapt.

Your family is not perfect. You are not perfect. You and the persons in your family respond to situations under the influence of each

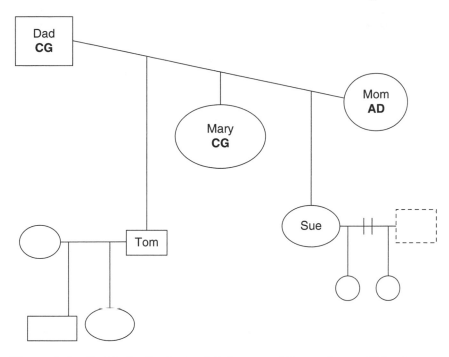

Figure 9.2   Smith family during Moderate and Severe Stage of Mom's Alzheimer's disease; Mary and Dad are CG (Caregivers).

member's personal choices, the emotional make-up of each person, and your common and unique formative experiences.

You may be an offspring of individuals who collapsed under stress. You may be someone with a parent who responded to stress with steely, emotionless thought and action. You may be part of a family that ordinarily rolls calmly with the punches. As someone close to a person with Alzheimer's, you know that there is a full range of ways that stress is handled among members of your caregiving family.

> *Ed's wife melted under the stress of caring for her beloved husband, as he went deeper and deeper into dementia. Some of their children simply lived in a state of denial. They did not believe that their father had anything wrong with him. On the other hand, some of their other children made a schedule for each week and were ever-present to help their mother.*

Whatever the range within your family, it is important for you to understand that your thinking, feeling, and acting under stress are influenced to some degree by the way your family thinks, feels, and acts. The better you can recognize what is occurring, the better you can make wise choices about your responses.

In your adult relationships with friends or with colleagues, you may have developed an ability to respond to stress situations without escalating anxiety or without shutting your feelings down or running away from things. You may find, however, that you do not do as well with stress within your family. You may be good at conflict resolution professionally or socially but not so good when you are back within a family situation.

> *Tom is a pastor known to listen well and respond gently and wisely. This is in sharp contrast to the way he deals with certain kinds of ongoing stresses in his own life. A well-loved uncle and mentor has lived with Tom and his wife for many years. The uncle's serious physical problems became compounded by growing dementia. Tom's responses at this time moved between long periods of silence broken by giving abrupt orders. He avoided all show of feelings when he and his wife faced difficult choices about how to live with the uncle's suffering.*
>
> *John and Ann are from very different families when it comes to conflict. Ann's family shouts and argues about everything and then all of them pull together. John grew up where there was rational discourse about everything and then the one in authority made the decision. The couple found a way to have a generally good marriage in their long life with each other. Ann is now moving from the Early-to-Mild to the Moderate Stage of Alzheimer's disease. John is having trouble dealing with Ann's extended family and some of his own children as they try to problem-solve how best to care for Ann.*

You are not a prisoner to family patterns. You don't need to repeat or react in your family style. You can discover options for yourself if you recognize and name both your personal style and your family patterns under stress. You can challenge yourself and say "No Way!" to an old thought pattern or an automatic reaction. You can choose to alter the way you meet a tense or painful situation. You can rejoice and be glad for the ways you or your family problem-solve under stress. You can choose to manage your patterns in the caregiving experience, so you don't lose yourself nor lose what you value in your family.

Joanna was a middle child in a large family. She was bright and creative and had a need to make "everything okay" for her family. She expended a lot of energy trying to make this happen. Her family came to depend on her to "fix" things, even though in the process they often had to put up with her anger, frustration, and manipulation of other family members. When her mother developed Alzheimer's, Joanna could not make everything right. In the face of losing their mother day by day to this disease, the family began to break apart with flaring tempers and quiet despair. Joanna's ways did not change things, and she had little heart to try. During the long Alzheimer's disease journey, Joanna owned that she was not responsible to do what she couldn't. She began to respect each of her brothers and sisters for handling the changes as best they could. She listened as much as she talked. She had to let herself receive help as well as give it.

Change is a major cause of stress and anxiety in all of life. Ongoing change is almost a definition of life for the person and family dealing with Alzheimer's disease. It can present the greatest pitfall for you. From beginning to end, you as caregiver are dealing with mental, emotional, and physical changes in the one suffering with the disease. What worked yesterday is not sufficient or it does not work today. You deal with changes in your own lifestyle. Your adjustment to the demands of caregiving has affected your job decisions. You can't move away or take certain work hours. Little by little, your patterns in social relationships change, pressured by time or fatigue. You and your family experience limits on some activities. Money, time, and patience challenges go up and down.

Sophie and Arthur were relatively young with three children when Arthur was diagnosed with Alzheimer's disease. Arthur was in his mid-fifties. Arthur was a well-known professional in the community whose job involved accounting procedures. The dementia made work impossible for Arthur, and he reacted with lots of anger toward members of his family, especially toward Sophie. He would sometimes strike Sophie and leave marks. His behavior was also unpredictable in public, so to protect Arthur and herself from embarrassment, Sophie chose to cut them off from almost all previous social activities and friendships. They became very isolated, and this did not end until Arthur was placed in a care facility.

Mary's friends and family encourage Mary to take a four-day weekend with her bridge club to have a timeout from her role as caregiver for her husband, Sam. The care facility sees Sam as stable. A daughter-in-law will be on vacation from work and will fill in. A neighbor volunteers to see Sam every day and call Mary if there are problems. Mary decides to go.

Three weeks before the trip, the care facility notifies Mary that they will be moving Sam to a different building, but they are not sure if it will be before or after her trip. The daughter-in-law fears she may have to cut her vacation short. The week of the trip, the neighbor thinks her children have been exposed to chicken pox. Solutions are proposed to deal with all the "maybes."

Mary cancels everything. She doesn't know or care if this is the wise thing to do. She is just fatigued by the ongoing struggle she feels in dealing with her thoughts, feelings, and actions during continuing change.

Change can become the enemy for the caregiver family that sets up a pretty hopeless battle. It may help you if you can come to terms, or at least to a neutral familiarity, with the general way change works. If you know and can expect the mental and emotional processes that change triggers in most human beings, then you can get a handle on how it works in you. If you can recognize what is happening in you when change happens, then you will be less anxious or powerless in facing it. The fact is that change can produce growth in you. It can help you grow. It is quite healthy to wish or pray in a given year that you will skip any possible opportunities for such growth. These prayers are not known to have any great success, however.

In fact, we can measure a child's learning and growth by watching the way he or she deals with change. Play and school are all about learning through facing new players and new realities. So, if change is so normal and even essential, why is it so tough? You can see the loss and pain it brings to you and the person with Alzheimer's disease. Can you avoid being overwhelmed and destroyed by this?

Much depends on the way you deal with change. Examine your patterns of response to change and see what works for you and what works against you. Evaluate your patterns and tools and decide what you need to strengthen and what you need to leave behind.

Here are some Guidelines for Stress Management:

1. Accept the change as real.

There are some situations when you cannot prevent change, and often that change means loss of something good. The change caused by dementia may be slow or fast. The person with dementia becomes different. The ways you relate to that person are modified. Your routine or practices become different. "That's the way it is now." Don't keep saying, "It shouldn't be this way." It just is the way it is.

> *One of the great pieces of advice that my mother gave me was, "Don't look back!!" She hated regret, and she strongly realized that one cannot reclaim the past. I am not certain that I fully understood this advice until I was much older. My mother was able to do all that she could at the moment, and then she was able to move ahead with the self-assurance that "I did all that I could, and I now must move forward to address the challenges of today."*

2. Know that change usually makes you feel uncomfortable.

You may feel lost, challenged, or confused. "Oh, he is different today. What am I feeling and how am I acting? What do I do about it? I hate this." Just don't choose to stay there.

Tom felt that he had lost a part of himself the first time his beloved wife Janet did not recognize him. He had already lost the security of her wise thoughts. He missed the way her humor and affection gave him comfort. He was afraid that if he really accepted that she sometimes did not know him, that he would have nothing. Tom felt rattled and fuzzy about himself as he lived with the "new."

3. Recognize that change gives you a new "normal."

You may hate it or adjust quickly to it, but you can recognize change. Take it for what it is. Come to terms with specific change but don't confuse it with "everything is changed." The sun still rises; the rain falls. You are you.

When the personality and recognizable style fades in the person with Alzheimer's, you don't have to lose everything about him. Don't make it all or nothing. When some patterns are modified, don't discard all patterns. Nurture what remains. Know that seeing and recognizing something new is not the only piece in the picture. Avoid leaving behind all that was there before. Don't just say, "Change controls my life now." Adapt in a way that retains what is possible, what remains in you and in the other. The decision to do this gives you back your appropriate sense of power.

Over their years together, Tom and Janet had created memories, a family, a history of exploring new ideas and interests and building friendships. Tom brought pictures and stories about what was happening in his life and that of their family and friends to Janet. Sometimes she responded and he caught her old smile. He began to build for them a daily routine of becoming aware of some new fact or book, person or place and telling her about it. He knew her love of art had built his; he knew she had grown through his sense of adventure. This was now their way of being "Tom and Janet."

4. Don't get lost when you don't know where to go.

Painful change can cause you to deny everything that is happening. You try to go back and capture the past before the change.

"If we all pretend that John is as he always was, he will become that again." Denial doesn't work for long unless you cut yourself off from facts and other people.

On the other hand, shocking change can cause you to throw out everything but the sickness of Alzheimer's. Memories, values, and other commitments seem not to be real. This is the stage of dealing with change that feels like nothing remains of the old. "This is the way life will be from now on. This illness is the only reality for me now." Hopelessness can come. Fixing on the new reality as a way to ease the stress of uncertainty can distort the whole of reality and cause extensive and unnecessary loss.

> *Elizabeth was an only child and saw only one option for herself when her mother began to decline very rapidly with dementia. She had to take care of her mother. She spent many, many hours with her mother, despite the needs of her husband and their marriage. When she was not with her husband, he was frustrated. When she came home to him, she was so worn down by her caregiver role, that both she and her husband were frustrated.*

Some confusion may reign in your feelings, thoughts, and actions during this period of adjusting to change. You may go back and forth between denial and giving up everything. During this time called "disequilibration" (or being on a mental teeter-totter), you will also have times when you seek to adjust to find a way to build on what you have. When you haven't yet found a way to rebalance things, it is best simply to walk with the questions, "to live your way into the answer."

It is easy in the course of this helplessness or confusion to put your anger or anxiety on someone or something that you can blame. It might be children or siblings not cooperating, a spouse's work hours, coworkers' bad habits, God's not listening to you, or the irritating behavior of the Alzheimer's patient. The ghosts of past strains on relationships with families are likely to resurface in times of stress. Being in touch with yourself and your emotions and thought processes will help you sort through things and respond freely in ways that fit who you are and what you choose to be in this difficult time.

The members of Eleanor's family started out dealing as well as could be expected with their mother's Alzheimer's. They were saddened, some denied, and then accepted what was happening. The members closest to her kept the other members updated on the changes and concerns. Basically, they were in it together.

Then, disturbing behaviors began. With each new loss or symptom, their togetherness fractured. They had as many ideas about what should be happening with her care as there were stars in the sky. Some read new articles on the disease and bombarded the others with expectations of how things should be done. Some just tried to deal with the moment. A couple became vigorously prayerful. One proclaimed continually that "No good God could let this happen." On occasion, a family member tried to give some leadership, but old rivalries about power and past mistakes resurfaced. Darkness and fear were real to them. They were losing their mother and their family. There was need for each family member to own his or her feelings and process the losses suffered. As each one could, they needed to reach out. They needed to do what they could for their mother and for each other.

5. Put together what remains of the old with what is present in the new.

Find ways to integrate what was and what is now. You may end up with 50 percent of the old and 50 percent of the new.

In going through the process of dealing well with change, you will find something new in yourself, something new in your life. It may be serenity, it may be wisdom, or it may be the comfort of being more aware and appreciative of who you are as a person. You may end up knowing something that you want to share with others in order to ease their growth. This process will take time. Occasionally, you may do it very quickly. Other times, it may go slowly and some changes may take a longtime until they are fully integrated.

Bob and Mary had been married a great many years when Mary was diagnosed with Alzheimer's disease. Bob was still employed, but Mary's condition caused him to consider carefully what was important to him. He decided that he would give up his job to give her care. He was mostly okay with this decision, for it solved a number of logistical issues. Mary died much sooner than expected, given the normal course of Alzheimer's, and Bob neither regretted his giving up his job nor the time that he got to spend with Mary. After her death, he returned to work.

John had always loved polka music. When he was young he played in a polka band. After John developed Alzheimer's, his son, Ernie, brought tapes of old time polka music and played them when he came to visit at the Care Center. After each piece he would ask his dad what he liked or didn't like about that piece. Ernie would write down what his dad said and read it to John if he wanted it. On following visits, Ernie would replay the favorite pieces and go through the process again with new pieces. John usually sparked up when music time came, and Ernie knew he was giving his father pleasure.

In the later stages of dealing with a change, push to recognize what is happening to integrate the old and the new. Know that it takes time and pain. Don't push too much too hard. If you are seeking to integrate too many changes at one time, it may just be overwhelming and you can't integrate anything well. Put some things on the backburner; don't forget them, just don't seek to handle everything at once. You cannot force healthy adaptation either by ignoring or by just pushing. When the integration does not come, walk patiently with the question. Ask yourself "Who do I want to be, and what do I want for the situation when this piece is integrated?"

Mary Ann and her husband Mike faced his growing dementia when he was in his late fifties. Their youngest son, Tom, was still in college. They both had extended family living in the area. It was not very long before Mike left work and went on disability. Family members provided some time to being in their home with Mike when Mary Ann was at work.

As Mike's Alzheimer's began to move out of the Early-to-Mild Stage into the Moderate Stage, Mary Ann faced the decision to cut her work to fewer hours so that she could work out of her home while she took care of Mike. Some extended family members began to have serious health problems of their own with concurrent financial problems. Tom wrestled with the decision to drop out of college altogether for a variety of reasons. A realtor friend suggested that Mary Ann look into selling her home and move into a smaller, more manageable space. Mary Ann felt completely overwhelmed and lonely without being able to count on Mike's wise counsel and support.

Mary Ann felt that she needed to take time to help Tom make a good decision about college. She had no choice but to integrate her new life of both working at home and caring for Mike. While she had great concern for what was going on in the extended family, she knew she could not put much time or energy into their concerns. The question of selling the house also had to be put on the back burner for the time being.

6. Expect more CHANGE.

Don't count on change being finished. Don't live with constant anxiety about the next change. Remember how you have faced and dealt with change successfully in the past. Recall past times when you tried to bypass it or give into pain and confusion. Recall what didn't work. Know that you can face it and handle it. Know that you don't have to like or welcome it. Know that you can survive and grow from it.

Teresa's two sons and daughter had interacted well together to face the changes necessary in her life because of worsening Alzheimer's disease. They rotated responsibilities around contact with medical consultants, financial matters, finding appropriate living and care settings, providing as much recreation and outside stimulation as Teresa's condition would allow. Three years into the journey with their mother, one son received a job promotion that would move him temporarily out of the country, and the daughter became aware of how much her husband and family resented the priority she was giving to "Grandma." All three faced the reality of the changes that they had not expected.

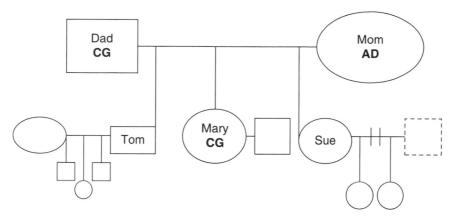

Figure 9.3   Smith family rebalanced stage of Alzheimer's disease.

In the face of the stress in your life because of Alzheimer's, you gain power back when you know what is going on and when you have tools to deal with it. You do not have much control over Alzheimer's disease. You can, however, take control over how you deal with the anxiety that comes when you recognize that change in your life and the life of the person for whom you care (Figure 9.3).

FROM GENERATION TO GENERATION

Rules, written and unwritten, are the legacy each of us carries with us from our background. When either very relaxed or very stressed, we will be inclined to repeat or react against what we learned when we didn't know we were learning it.

Healthy caregivers know what's in the baggage they carry into their world of caregiving. This book adds many levels of "to do's" and "not to do's." There are recommendations, suggestions, and bits of useful information to inform your decisions and actions as a caregiver. Unique to the puzzle that is your life, however, are layers of rules that came long before you became a caregiver. You formed these rules from your life experiences, your education, your belief system, your personality style, and from the things that came with being part of the families you chose and the family into which you were born. It is to the rules that come from family messages that we will discuss now.

All of us tend to repeat or to react against the personal rules we bring as baggage into our current lives. It can be helpful to pay attention to how you came to the rules you choose to follow and the impact they have on you today.

If you grew up in a family like mine, you would know that whining or complaining was the most unforgivable behavior in a family member. "Quit whining." "Stop your belly-aching!" was the home-made phrase. I like to whine, and I often thought, "Someday I will come back to this family, and I will whine and whine and no one can stop me." As an adult, as a professional, as a friend, what can I not tolerate in others? Whining, of course! When someone whines about something to me, I have to force myself to stop and repeat silently, "He is not a moral degenerate; he is just whining." Under stress or when I am relaxed, I still can act as if I believe people who whine need to be told to "Grow up!"

My friend Josh grew up in a family where everybody shouted when they were excited. They expressed every feeling they ever had, and they seemed not to listen to one another. He hated it. When he married and had his own family, no one was ever allowed to raise a voice to another and from his point of view, the fewer feelings anyone expressed, the better life was for everybody. He is as much controlled by his family message by reacting against it as I am by repeating mine.

What are/were the spoken and unspoken rules on giving care for the ill in your family? How far back do they go? Who accepts them and who rejects them?

I remember distinctly walks with my great-grandmother. She was a very spry woman, and even though she lived until I was 17, she always conceived of me as a child. She loved to parade me through her neighborhood, and not only was it a time to show me off, but it was also a time to share important lessons. One teaching moment that I remember always occurred in front of the same house. Gram would stop and say to me, "That is where Sarah lived. She never got married. She stayed with her parents and took care of them until they died." As a male and a child, this lesson did not have much meaning to me, until I began to watch my own mother relating to her mother. I believe my mother felt guilty for marrying and moving a thousand miles away. Whenever my grandmother would tell my mother that she was ill, my mother ran to her side. I once asked my grandmother what it was like when my mother married my father, and my grandmother, without hesitation, said, "She left me!!" The intergenerational message clearly valued daughters living with and caring for their parents.

Gail and Barb both grew up in families in which men were conditioned to believe that it is "women's work" to care for family member who are ill. They have innumerable female friends who have expressed frustration and outrange at their brothers who do not do their fair share of caregiving for aging parents. My friend, Gail, recently shouted with frustration at the fact that her brother, who lives in the same town as their mother, still expects Gail to shoulder the responsibility of medical care for the mother, even though Gail lives six hours away from them. And, just last week, Barb expressed anger with her brother who expects Barb to manage their mother's needs while the mother is in a nursing home. Both Barb and her brother live in the town where their mother is, but the brother involves himself only to check on how Barb thinks the mother is doing.

What are/were the rules about asking for help? Is it easier to ask a family member than an outsider? Is outside help a sign that family members don't care enough?

Many years ago, I started a support group for family members of Alzheimer's victims. Even though the group met in mid-town, I simply could not understand why African-Americans never joined the group. I began to ask my African-American friends if they knew anyone with Alzheimer's disease, and to a person, they told me that they did not. I found that very strange until I engaged a couple of Africa-American pastors in conversation about the absence. They told me that in their

*congregations, there were strong "rules" in families govern-
ing getting outside help and even stronger rules about keeping older persons in the homes of their family until death.
Recently, when discussing care of elders with an African-
American counselor, she echoed the pastors' perception by
stating, "We would never utilize a nursing home. We take
care of our people at home."*

Do you have any rules that come with the complications of blended
families? How do you check out expectations and perceptions?

*My dear aunt, Sade, is 87 years old, and she struggles with the
mental deterioration that accompanies Alzheimer's disease.
Nearly 50 years ago, she divorced her first husband with whom
she had a son, George. She has been married to her present husband, John, for more than 20 years. Sade is confused about many
things, and she and her husband live out in the country. George,
her only child, lives several states away from his mother, and he
is frustrated by Sade's husband's inability or unwillingness to
discuss the situation with him. John acts as though the responsibility for Sade's care lies with her son and not with her husband.
When approached by her son, the husband simply says, "I cannot talk about it, right now." That begins and ends the conversation. The husband is unable or unwilling to arrange appropriate
care for Sade, and that frustrates her son. Of course, George
conceptualizes this as part of the ongoing strain of the fact that
he is John's stepson. John has never had other children, so dealing with an adult stepson is difficult. Recently, circumstances
have begun to convince John that he and George need to cooperate and do what is best for Sade.*

People do recognize times when rules that have worked well are
no longer working and have to change. Can you recognize "seasons"
within your own life and the lives of family members when attitudes
and roles no longer fit?

*Ted was always the witty, independent, and somewhat aloof
member of the family. He was second oldest and remembers*

looking back from the front seat of the family station wagon at all the "little kids" clamoring for attention in the back. He recalls telling himself, "I'd better learn to look out for myself because no one is going to have time to do it for me."

The family rule was that Ted would go it alone. He has done reasonably well in life while marching to his own drummer. Now, as his mother is moving from the Early-to-Mild Stage to Moderate Stage of Alzheimer's disease and his father's health is seriously failing, he finds himself the only one of his siblings living in the same area as his parents. To the amazement of his siblings, Ted has stepped forward and begun to organize the family on how to care for their parents. He and his wife have invited his parents to move into a mother-in-law apartment in their home. He has taken leadership with his father on the next steps for them.

WHEN ENOUGH IS ENOUGH

Accept that which you cannot change; change that which you can; be wise enough to know the difference.

The ever-changing mobile of your family is unique. It has many layers that impact who you are as an individual and as a caregiver. It provides patterns that you automatically or deliberately repeat or react against as you deal with the continual changes that Alzheimer's brings to your life. The normal process of dealing with that change can create a serious pitfall but you can learn to deal with it wisely. On the other hand, regardless of the skill and awareness that you have in being a caregiver with a family, there are times when "enough is enough."

Being powerless can be the worst and most destructive of stressors. Beating your head endlessly against an unmoving wall achieves nothing. Generally, it becomes extreme frustration or despair. Can you recognize when you need to acknowledge that you are hanging on to an expectation or a hope when you need to let go?

I have to stop wanting and waiting for my brothers to volunteer a more active role in caring for mom's needs. I will "reframe" my expectations and send them a list of responsibilities that need to be assumed among us when we meet next week.

Uncle Charlie's behavior around the house is becoming more bizarre, and my daughters are embarrassed to bring their friends home. My husband, John, keeps telling me how grateful he is that I can take care of his uncle in our home. I am exhausted from all the care that Charlie needs. Because I handle my part-time job by phone and computer here at home, I feel that I should do what my family has done for generations and 'take care of our own.' It's not working. I'm coming to believe that it would be much wiser if John and I found an affordable care facility for Uncle Charlie.

Ethel came often to the care facility where her beloved George lived. One day, she took him for a ride, and upon their return, he asked her if she would like to come in to meet his wife. This was a real blow to Ethel, for it signaled the first time that George did not recognize her as his wife. Ethel, the consummate caregiver, accepted the invitation and accompanied George inside. He was confused when he could not find his wife, but Ethel was very thoughtful and excused herself, leaving his room. A couple of minutes later, she returned to his room, and he greeted her as his wife, wondering where she had been. He did not mention the other woman whom he wanted to introduce to his wife. Ethel just rolled with his state of mind at the moment. She would cry later but she was ready to act first on George's reality.

Reflection:

- When you need to re-evaluate expectations about your role as caregiver, do you have some independent "sounding board?" Do you need one? What criteria do you use to know when "enough is enough"? Which expectations are most difficult for you to judge well? Your own? Those of family? Those of the one for whom you care?
- Do you believe that working successfully with the needs of others requires the ability "to care and not to care?" What

does the balance look like for you when you both 1) invest yourself personally in another's need and, at the same time, 2) give yourself the distance of knowing this person is not you and you need to set the other person's burden down at times? What keeps you from giving yourself such appropriate distance?

- When have you been most successful "agreeing to disagree with others," especially in spoken and unspoken family messages about decisions or expectations? Can you still do this for yourself even if the other does not "agree to "disagree"?

- Have you experienced any "burn out," losing sense of self as an individual, or negative changes in personality? A time when you did not recognize that "enough is enough"?

GRIEF AND LOSS AND ITS IMPACT ON CAREGIVERS

Grief is an experience that allows one to deal with the change of loss. In your "long good-bye" to the one suffering with Alzheimer's, your grief as a caregiver is often ignored or misunderstood, even by you. There are things about your continuing losses in the Alzheimer's journey that are both different from and like other grieves in your life. There are unique and common ways that you can do grief work or avoid it. As basic a reality as grief is, it can be a pitfall in your role as caregiver if you do not understand and recognize what grief looks like as a piece of your Alzheimer's caregiving puzzle.

GRIEF WHEN YOU STILL HAVE THE PERSON YOU ARE LOSING

Grief for the family or caregivers of one with Alzheimer's disease is, first of all, a paradox. Paradox happens when two opposite things are true in your life at the same time. You are mourning your loss, while the person you are mourning stands in front of you.

So, grieving the big losses and the small losses with Alzheimer's means acknowledging that losses are happening. At precisely the same time, it means nurturing the life that remains. It means finding joy in the present moment and acknowledge a past that is gone and a future that is uncertain. Such paradoxes can create confusion and questions: Doesn't one side of the paradox cancel out the other? How can both exist for you in an honest and healthy way? They just do. In fact, experiencing grief as a juggling of opposite feelings and facts is normal and essential in your situation. You, as a caregiver, have two opposite and equal realities to handle as you grieve. It is a unique challenge, and most caregivers can do it well, whether they recognize it or not. Acknowledging what you are doing, however, can help you affirm both the challenges you face and your strength in facing them.

John felt that some days he both loved and hated his wife, Jane. He would do anything for her, even though he believed it would be better for her and everyone else if she could just fall asleep one night and never wake up. He was sad when he remembered the things he no longer could do in his career because of his role as primary caregiver. He was angry with other family members who seemed to leave him alone to carry the burden. On the other hand, he resented them when they acted as if they could care for her as well as he could. After all, he and Jane knew and loved each other as no one else could.

Suzie and Judy never talked about it, but both felt that they would be unfaithful and not loving of their father if they accepted that he was really lost to them with his dementia. Suzie, "Daddy's little girl," believed that real fidelity would mean she kept fighting the facts, because "I will not let this happen to him." Judy feared facing the future because she felt that it was her responsibility as the oldest to keep the family together after dad died and she didn't know if she could do it. So long as he was alive, his presence would keep things together. The family doctor knew them well and asked them to talk about the fact that their father's disease was terminal. He asked them to share all their feelings so that they could make realistic decisions about their dad's care.

THE CYCLE OF GRIEF

Ordinary grief is not just one feeling or thought. It is a process of dealing with the loss through which you pass. Each person handles it differently, but there are common stages. The change or loss happens, and you are shocked and may deny that it is happening. When the shock wears off or the denial cannot be continued, you acknowledge that the change or loss is real. Feelings of anger, of being abandoned or betrayed or treated unjustly can take control. You may try to find a way to-change-the-change or loss. You think about and seek to try any way that could turn things around. Such attempts are followed by sadness or depression because of what is gone. This time of feeling the loss is part of the "work" of the grief process. You move out of this depression into an acceptance that you have suffered a loss. You integrate the loss into the bigger picture of "how does life function now?" This integration is not the same as becoming resigned to the facts. It goes beyond resignation to the acceptance that life does continue, and you will make yourself a part of that ongoing life. This is the work of the normal grief process.

> *The other day, I met a friend at church. I had not seen him for a while, and he wanted to tell me about his struggles with his wife's health. They have been married for over fifty years. Three years ago, his wife began experiencing the signs and behaviors of Alzheimer's disease. He and their children were able to care for her in their home, but seven months ago, the decision was made to place her in a care facility. He said that it has been a very hard seven months for him, but he has adjusted. He visits her each day, but he also has found a job that has given him a new lease on life. At the age of eighty, he goes to work each day, but his supervisor has told him, "Come in when you want and leave when you want." He is working through the daily demands of the grief process, but he has diversions that have helped him move ahead.*

No two people grieve alike. Perhaps, no two losses in your own life are worked through in exactly the same way. A step in the process may take weeks or months or it may be completed in days or hours. You may go backwards and forwards in the steps of the process. The constant fact, however, is that you cannot jump over the process of grieving change or loss that matter to you. You cannot ignore or go under grief; you cannot fly over it or around it. You must do the "work of grief" if you are to deal with the change of loss. Unresolved grief tends to remain or come back and get in the way of being truly alive in the next moment. You can get "stuck" in a stage or process of grief.

> *Herm's wife, Marie, developed dementia after 40 years of marriage, and Herm finally decided to place her in a care facility. He became consumed with grief and remained stuck in the grief process, even after she died. One indication of being stuck was the great resentment that he felt for others who were able to celebrate their fiftieth wedding anniversaries. Herm refused to attend these celebrations, and he openly admitted that he would not go, because he and Marie had been unable to celebrate theirs.*

There are added factors that can complicate the grief process and some of them are very common in the grief of those giving care for a loved one with Alzheimer's disease.

- One loss often involves multiple related losses. At a certain stage of Alzheimer's disease, the caregiver juggles the grief of many things involved with a new loss. Your loved one may not always remember who you are and who he or she is. With this, a level of companionship and intimacy is gone for you; other family members are numbed or profoundly hurt by this new change; the part-time work in your chosen job or career is less and less possible with the need to give more constant care. There is more frustration and anxiety in your loved one and you become aware that you have no power to relieve your loved one's confusion. Some of these losses blend into one another. Some are so sharp as to need a separate grieving process. You will take just one moment at a time, grieve what you can and know that there will be a time for what is on the back burner.

- The losses can go on and on. When one loss is integrated into what life has become, another is at the door step. Fatigue, numbness, and pressures can build up. It is important, but difficult, to stay in the present. As much as possible, do the ordinary things: eat, sleep, exercise, laugh, tell stories, watch a distracting show, or call a friend who always knows the gossip.

- The grieving process of others impacts you. Some people on whom you counted may leave you alone because they cannot bear the losses which you share. Some expect you to care for them in their grief as well as to care for the patient and yourself. Some are stuck in stages of grief, denial, anger, bargaining, or depression. They know you can't do their work for them. Yet, being with them can be a great burden.

Margaret was a valued friend of Don and Angie, but when Don's Alzheimer's disease made his behavior unpredictable, Margaret stopped coming to see her friend Angie. Margaret was married to John, and she freely told Angie that she did not want to visit, because in Don and Angie she saw her future self, a caregiver for a person with dementia. In reality, John was not showing any signs or symptoms of dementia, but in her mind, Margaret was afraid of what the future might hold for her, and she did not want to see that in her friend, Angie.

SPECIAL CIRCUMSTANCES FOR THE ALZHEIMER'S CAREGIVER

There are some realities that need special mention if you are to provide yourself with the information you need as an Alzheimer's caregiver dealing with loss and grief.

- There are probably no rituals for you to use to mark the losses you are experiencing. No graduations, no series of wakes or funerals as you move through one stage to another. There are usually no blessings or toasts or recognized signs of loss that you can share with others or use to affirm your feelings or transitions. This can make it harder for you to own your grief and let it be legitimate. It is good for some to write, or draw, or create their own rituals, alone or with others.

A local hospital sponsors a monthly "Express Yourself Through the Arts." It is a Saturday program for people experiencing loss, and it is done with the help of local artists who help those attending create something. Many of the attendees are experiencing an illness, but some are there to celebrate a loved one who is in a slow decline in health. In talking to participants, they report that this is an opportunity to get out, to do something fun, and to dedicate their project to their loved one.

- The grieving process of the Alzheimer's caregiver is often overlooked or minimized by others or themselves. Sometimes this is because you, the caregiver, are too busy giving care. Sometimes this is because you are involved in a paradoxical response which requires you to grieve a loss and invest in a new response at the same time. Sometimes this is because some people in your world do not value a person with dementia enough to affirm their loss. Often it is simply because there are so many losses that you as a caregiver must absorb in the course of the Alzheimer's disease that no loss along the way is recognized. Because the losses experienced have no clear beginning or clear ending, it may never seem like an appropriate time to stop and grieve. Remember, for you as caregiver, it is not only appropriate for you to recognize grief during the process but also to let yourself acknowledge it and work it through. It may take a few seconds or a more extended time.

Lucille was always in a hurry. She lived next door to me when I was a child, and she seemed to be constantly running from one task to another. She hardly ever slowed down, and at one point, we kids would repeat the lines from Alice in Wonderland when we would see her: "I'm late, I'm late for a very important date.

No time to say 'hello' 'good-bye'; I'm late, I'm late, I'm late!!"
Her approach to life did not change when her husband, Ted,
was diagnosed with Alzheimer's disease. Lucille rushed around
as she always had, caring for Ted, but not caring for herself.
She denied the grieving process, and as Ted's condition contin-
ued to deteriorate, Lucille found herself becoming ill and not
able to care for Ted. A skilled and thoughtful physician helped
Lucille recognize the damage she was doing to herself and pro-
vided assistance to help her slow down and look after herself.

• The long-term of the Alzheimer's journey can create overlooked and hidden emotions in the caregiver, such as perva-
sive depression or anxiety. Because there is always another
"shoe to fall" or more loss to absorb, you as the caregiver can
get into a negative mode of response that seems to become
"natural." Family, friends, support group members, and professionals working in the caregiving process need to be alert
to such changes in the caregiver and intervene, if possible.
You, as caregiver, need to cultivate the friends and interactions
that can help you identify negative changes in this direction.

Faye and her husband, Howard, lived in a small town. They
had many friends and five children. The small town was not a
place that any of their children found fulfilling, so the children
scattered to larger communities where they found work. When
Howard was diagnosed with dementia, Faye had the insight to
know that she, too, was vulnerable to all of the physical and
emotional demands of caregiving. She had read of the dangers,
and she was determined to balance her life, so she would not
experience unnecessary illnesses. She carefully reached out to
six of her closest friends in the community, and she arranged
with them a weekly outing. She asked her friends to bear with
her when she was grieving and to refuse to let her make excuses
for not attending their weekly outings. She also asked them to
be true friends. She asked that they be honest in telling her
what they were seeing each week in her. Faye structured a
once-a-week meeting with dear friends as a social outlet, as

well as a time for honest comments from others. Today, Faye believes that her friends and their caring comments, while not easy to hear, saved her from many of the consequences of long-term caregiving.

THE "TO DO" LIST FOR A CAREGIVER DEALING WITH GRIEF

Pace Yourself

- You may find yourself on an emotional roller-coast of loss and hope.
- Be honest and aware of your losses and the thoughts and emotions you have.
- Don't try to deal with them all at once.

Take Time Out

- It is good and wise to "turn off" your feelings and thoughts concerning your losses for a time.
- Take time out from caregiving to take care of you. Attend to your needs and grief. Take 20 minutes a day with a cup of coffee or tea (or something else) to process your losses and take care of yourself. Daydream or just "be."

Have a Goal

- Know that you need to deal with grief in an ongoing way. Name your goal for dealing with grief and growth. *I will do more than survive grief and loss. I will find a way to thrive over time.*
- Do a regular check-up on "where am I stuck in my grieving process?" Where am I strong?

Never Believe "One Size Fits All"

- Know that no two persons grieve alike. Don't expect family and friends to deal with Alzheimer's and caregiving in exactly the same way you do. Know that they will not always agree with or support you. Don't take responsibility for their thoughts or feelings.

Build on Your Strengths

- Check out your spirituality and how you understand life. Let your spirit be strengthened by what you value and believe. Put your caregiving in the "Big Picture" of life. How is loss, grief, and change a part of this picture for you?

Reach out

- Trust in yourself. Trust in your faith or value system. Trust in your ability to reach out to friends, professionals, and support groups for help in dealing with your loss and with your growth. A growing body of literature and scholarship is being devoted to the Alzheimer's patients and you, the caregiver.

Regret: The Guilt in Caregivers

- Nobody is perfect. Chances are that you are not an exception to this in your role as caregiver. You may judge yourself as guilty of not being "good enough" in what you do. You may recognize simple regrets or serious feelings of guilt. It is important that you can understand and evaluate your areas of regret and areas of guilt so that you address them appropriately and wisely. Caregiving for a person with dementia over significant periods of time can be full of new learning, stresses, fatigue, and frustrations. It is a time ripe with potential for mistakes as well as growth opportunities. Take time to reflect on what you know, understand, and feel about "Regret" and "Guilt." Learn to recognize the difference between guilt and regret as you desire to improve or change as you give care.

Appropriate Guilt and Inappropriate Guilt

- All guilt is not equal. There are measures by which you can evaluate if what you are feeling is appropriate or not.
- Appropriate guilt occurs when what you did was a serious wrong, you knew it was wrong, and you did it anyway. "I should have or should not have done this thing; I knew it and I deliberately did it anyway." Serious wrong requires ownership of it, repentance of it, amendment (making it right),

forgiving self, and moving on. Avoiding or refusing to deal with appropriate Guilt creates a burden for a psychologically healthy person. Dealing with Guilt allows you to grow and move on.

- Inappropriate Guilt is not healthy. It creates in you feelings and responses that do not fit or resolve the feelings. Inappropriate Guilt occurs when that which you did was not a serious matter, or you did not know it was serious, or you did not choose to do it—knowing it was serious. The appropriate evaluations for such an action is "I wish I had done that. I regret that I did that." Such a response can lead to appropriate sadness, embarrassment, regret, and moving on.

- Holding on to an inappropriate Guilt or trying to treat it as if it were appropriate can be harmful to you. You can turn it inward, and it can become depression. On the other hand, you can turn it outward as anger or confusion. You do not really get past inappropriate Guilt if you mislabel it and handle it as appropriate Guilt.

Tom often called and visited his father in the nursing home. The nursing home staff phoned one afternoon to tell Tom that his father had been asking for him. They saw no immediate crisis but suggested that he touch base with his dad soon. Because he had a long scheduled business meeting out of town, Tom decided to wait until he was back the following evening when he would be free to have a longer visit with his father. Tom's dad died unexpectedly the next afternoon. Tom beat himself up with inappropriate Guilt until he learned to say to himself, "It's not that I should have gone back because I knew my dad was dying. If I had known that I would have gone instantly. The fact is I wish with all my heart I had gone to see him that night." Regret is much more honest and fitting than Guilt, and it helps Tom bring honest closure to his feeling

Sources of Regret and Guilt

Among caregivers there are some common sources that lead to feelings of regret and Guilt. There are also common sources of mixing-up appropriate and inappropriate Guilt. Again, reflection and understanding can lead to responses that fit.

Perfectionist Tendencies

- The expectation that you should be able to do things perfectly could be a view that you as caregiver bring to your role. On the other hand, it may be the one for whom you are caring, the rest of family or outsiders who expect all things to be done without mistake. This may be an old family message, it may be a part of your spirituality, or it may just be your personality. When things do not go perfectly, you can assume Guilt, rather than Regret. You need to challenge that expectation and say, "I wish it had been different than it was" when that fits the situation. Avoid, "I should have been different than I was" unless you have all the proper ingredients for Guilt. If you continually accept demands of perfection from yourself or others, you can run out of energy, humor, or self-esteem. The "perfect" can become the enemy of the "good."

The Unknowns

- First-time caregivers, as well as experienced caregivers, face changes and doing things "for the first time" over and over. The person suffering from dementia may follow a pattern but is always uniquely himself or herself. "Dealing with the unexpected" means you will sometimes get-it-right and sometimes you will not. If you take on inappropriate Guilt, you can become anxious and fearful of the unexpected rather than learning "to go with the flow."

Past Issues

- Unresolved conflict between you and the person for whom you are caring can cause endless inappropriate Guilt. If the person with Alzheimer's disease is in a position to resolve the conflict, you may want to try to do so. Otherwise, you will want to do your own work to set it aside and deal with what is happening today. If you find yourself acting out old patterns or angers rather than dealing with today's issues, name that and own Guilt if it is appropriate. Then, get yourself some help if it is needed and move on. If there are family patterns or messages, choose whether you want to repeat or reject them. Be the caregiver you want to be. If others, including the one for whom you are caring, insist on repeating these patterns, you may tell them what is happening and continue to act out of your own choices.

Personality Traits

- Own yourself. If you have a temper and it sometimes controls you, admit it; learn ways to manage it (Time Outs, good self-care, group support, seeking help). Own your Guilt or Regret, as is appropriate and move on. If you have a sharp tongue, learn to bite it sometimes. Learn humor, not sarcasm. If you fail, get up and start over. Don't let your style harm others over and over.

Lack of Affirmation

- Lack of appreciation can become pretty old. Recognize that for what it is. Learn to have reasonable expectations. Tell people your expectations. "A thank you would be nice." Put yourself in some settings of friends or support groups of people who know what it is to deal with situations like yours. Turn to your spirituality and to your humor. Deal appropriately with your Regret or Guilt so that you can "like" yourself and "affirm" yourself.

THE "TO DO" LIST FOR CAREGIVERS: DEALING WITH "GUILT" OR "REGRET"

Expect Some "Guilt" or "Regret"

- Unless you are unconscious or conscious but doing nothing, you will have things that you regret or about which you feel guilty. Deal with them when they happen. Back track and deal with them if they are in the past but impacting your caregiving role and skills at the present.

Make Honest Assessments

- You are not being fair or honest if you see every mistake or breakdown in your attitude or behavior as "appropriate Guilt." Check family patterns, the reasonableness of your expectations of yourself, and your judgments about the expectations others have of you and the skills you have for caregiving through the long and changing journey of caring for a person with Alzheimer's disease.

- You may not be honest or fair if you don't own appropriate responsibility when you do something wrong or harmful and you know what it is and you chose to do it anyway. Chalk it up to denial, to arrogance, to blaming somebody else for "making you do it." Whatever causes you to see no "shadow side" of yourself, get over it. Own your Guilt, deal with it appropriately, and move on.

Choose to Grow

- You don't have to grow from your mistakes, but chances are you will be more alive, more free, and happier if you do. Learn from what you have done, let your awareness change you in ways that are good for you. Don't become fearful, defensive, or unwilling to try again and start over.
- Spend some quiet time regularly taking care of yourself. Checking out what you are learning about your strengths and weakness. Own your "light" as well as your "shadow." Healthy self-esteem is an invaluable asset to the busy caregiver. Know your strengths and rejoice in them, or at least smile at them. Know your weaknesses, your challenges, and know that you can work with them.

Face Change and Avoid Harmful Patterns or Behaviors

- When it comes to doing harm to another, especially the one for whom you are providing care, be tough on yourself. Give yourself no lee-way in your efforts to get beyond and repair any such patterns or behaviors.

Be Glad When a New Piece of Your "Puzzle" Comes into Place

- Learn to identify and avoid "Potential Personal Pitfalls" as you continue to live in the unique Alzheimer's caregiving puzzle that is your life.
- Your time in caregiving is a key part of your life. Attend to your experience.

CHAPTER 10

Keeping Your Head Up

Janaan Manternach

TO LET GO OF DENIAL BRINGS PEACE AND WISDOM

Prior to the relationship that happens between an Alzheimer's individual and a caregiver are the experiences of denial and discovery. There's a hidden component in both that often occurs in the individual before it becomes apparent to others.

This is how it occurred between Carl and me. He would work too long on a talk that he had to give. I would go into his office and ask him why he was working so hard on something that he could have given without any preparation. I also found myself reminding him of appointments, but neither of us were concerned about that.

Carl began to ask me to do talks by myself that we were scheduled to give together. Again, I didn't think too much of that because they were topics that I could easily handle on my own. However, one evening when he was doing something that he did automatically every evening after dinner—take the garbage out to the can in the back of the house—something significant happened. I was putting the dishes in the dishwasher and suddenly I realized he was gone too long. I went out onto the patio and found Carl standing motionless with the garbage at his feet. He was obviously troubled, and I said, "It's okay! It's okay!" I picked up the bag and deposited it in the garbage can. He was still standing on the patio when I returned and when we got back into the house he looked at me and said, "I'm losing my mind!" We both knew the time of denial was over, and a major discovery had been made. We held each other and cried. That cry was a most unforgettable moment of acceptance and healing. But that is not the end of the story. As long as Carl wanted to and could carry the garbage bags, we took them out to the can together.

About the talks Carl asked me to give, the talks that were scheduled for us to give together, we continued to give them TOGETHER. I spoke but he assisted with the slides, set up the slide projector, turned the lights on and off, and made sure that I had the books and other materials I was using when I needed them. It was such a carefully concerted effort the audience scarcely noticed and seemingly didn't care that I was the only one who spoke.

When denial is happening in a family there are often clear enough signals but no one—NO ONE—neither the person with dementia nor those of us who will be affected want to believe it's happening. And although, today, we're far more open about the disease, there's still some stigma connected to it—if not in the minds of others—in our own minds.

CAREGIVING BECOMES AN ART WHEN WISDOM RESULTS IN KINDNESS

For many who eventually find themselves in the role of caregiver it does not come easily or naturally. I know from experience that I was unwilling, at first, to deal with what was happening in Carl. For example, one of the first signs that this role could become a life changer for me was the morning Carl could not put on his shoes. I was determined that he would and when he tried again, he put them on the wrong feet. This angered me. I roughly slipped them off his feet and told him to put them on right. He couldn't and for a period of time that morning I wouldn't. I painfully realized that my selfishness was going to be a real problem for both of us.

From being unable to put on his shoes, he was soon unable to dress himself and I became angry at both myself and him. I didn't want to be a caregiver; I felt that I simply couldn't. On the other hand, I loved him too much to abandon him and with that realization something palpable started to happen in me. As that movement began to take hold, I gradually became willing to care.

It was never all that easy but I know from years of experience that the Divine in us is powerful. We grow, by degrees, from being selfish to unselfish; we experience, at times, surprising glimpses of the nobler parts of ourselves; we slowly learn to make large allowances for another's dependence eclipsing our independence; we learn how to truly love another unconditionally. Mostly unaware of what is happening within, we become "graciously different."

TO GIVE UP ONE'S INDEPENDENCE IS, PERHAPS, THE MOST ENNOBLING EXPERIENCE FOR A CAREGIVER

This, like many other happenings with an Alzheimer's patient, occurs gradually. One of the first things that eroded my independence took awhile to happen. For almost a year, I could go to lunch with a friend or do other errands and leave Carl at home by himself. I always told him where I was going and approximately how long I'd be gone. That freedom ended abruptly one day when I returned and found him standing by the door. He was agitated and told me how worried he was. He kept asking me where I had been, and no amount of explaining seemed to help. From then on, I took him with me wherever I went or got someone to stay with him. That put serious limits on my independence but, amazingly, I accepted the change without any feelings of animosity. When this happens, it's a sign, often unnoticed, that a deeper acceptance of the disease has occurred. As a caregiver, we have grown.

The next major loss, which I name "shadowing," took place shortly thereafter. Carl wanted to be everywhere that I was. If I was working at my computer, he would stand by it until I would tell him to go somewhere else. Then he'd move only a few feet away. Gradually, it dawned on me that his aloneness with himself made my presence necessary. I then placed his favorite rocking chair near my computer and when I did that I noticed he wasn't only interested in being near me but also in what I was doing. I began telling him what I was doing, he read and remarked on it, and a new coworking relationship happened. This met his need and was a surprising help to me.

This need to be where he could see me grew and was exhibited in numerous ways. He'd follow me into the kitchen, the bedroom, the living room, the laundry room, and even the bathroom. At first, I found this hardly tolerable but gradually I became okay with it, so much so, that I'd invite him to go with me wherever I was going. Mysteriously, one day this need in him stopped, but by this time I was caught in its web. I needed to be where he was.

The next loss was harder for me than it might be for some. I always liked to go places with very little notice and could get ready quickly. This changed radically when Carl could no longer dress himself. It sometimes took longer than I expected because I could never gauge exactly how long it would take to get him ready. Sometimes it was harder for him to cooperate; sometimes it was easier. And, sometimes, he would panic and tell me he couldn't go where we were going.

Carl panicked one morning when we were flying back to Arlington, Virginia, from Dubuque, Iowa. I literally had to coax, beg, and guide him, step by step, into the car that took us to the airport and then into the terminal. He kept holding back and saying that he couldn't go. Members of my family assisted me which helped greatly. The agents at the airport were also helpful and by the time we boarded the plane he was fine. I was worried about what might happen when we got to Chicago and had to board another plane but all went smoothly. And when he saw the friends who were waiting for us when we arrived, he was overjoyed and completely over the panic he had struggled with so painfully when we started the trip. That, however, was the last trip that we took alone. From then on trips anywhere, even to Dubuque, Iowa, to be with family, required an additional ticket for someone to help me with Carl. But we continued, for a long time, going where we wanted to go.

The loss of independence can be one of the most destructive for a caregiver. It can cause anger, feelings of hopelessness, and even an erosion of self-worth. Fortunately, for me, I had friends who supported me enough that I could accept most of what happened as Carl became more and more dependent and I became less and less independent. It also forced me to be creative in nurturing what remained in him and exercising that together.

THE VIRTUE OF KINDNESS GROWS AS WE WILLINGLY ADJUST

Adjusting becomes the name of the game for us who are care or "sharegivers." This is not as easy as it may seem. In many instances you may feel an inner pull against a change that has to be made. You also may not see an apparent solution. Don't worry! A solution will dawn on you as you're falling asleep or meditating or cleaning up after a meal. In that moment, you'll recognize what has to be done. During that feeling of relief, you'll experience a surge of energy. Your spirit will be refreshed.

When Carl could no longer dress himself in the morning, I would get up first, take a shower and dress. Then I'd get him up, help him shower, and dress but by the time I was finished doing that I was perspiring and in need of another shower. Suddenly, it dawned on me that I should get him up first, help him shower, get him dressed, and have him sit in a comfortable chair while I took care of getting myself ready for the day. It was a perfect solution, an easy adjustment and, best of all, it made me feel kinder toward him.

Although an adjustment to almost every challenge is available, there are some challenges that belie that truth. At times a caregiver will find him or herself crying or wailing aloud. There is no sound as hollow as a cry that wells up from hopelessness. In several instances this happened to me.

One morning, we were about to leave for an appointment and were at the car. I opened the door on the passenger side and motioned to Carl to get in. He stood there. I kept begging him to get in and he continued to simply stand there. At 5'3", I was unable to lift him. He wasn't overweight but he was 6 foot tall. I realized painfully that if we didn't get on the way soon we'd be late for the appointment, and I would have to cancel it. When we got back into the house, he sat down in his favorite chair unaware of what had just occurred. I sat at our dining room table and wept. Then the thought struck me. I had to try to prepare Carl. And I did. Fifteen minutes before we were to leave I'd sit down with him and tell him where we were going, what we were going to do there, and how long we'd be gone. Then I'd tell him that he'd have to get into the car even though it might be hard for him. I would ask him if he thought he could and he always said, "Yes." Mysteriously, it worked. And although there were real moments of hesitation, he always did it. I would thank him with a hug because I needed him to do it and because he did it I was genuinely grateful. It was one of those moments of wisdom when I truly nurtured what remained.

This same phenomenon occurred on Sunday mornings when it was time to go to Mass. He somehow sensed when I dressed him in a suit and tie that we were going someplace that he didn't want to go. I solved that with the help of friends. They would come over and were strong enough to coax and lift him from his chair and help him into their car.

It was a peaceful solution which we celebrated every Sunday morning after Mass by going to Carl's favorite restaurant for brunch. Mysteriously, when we arrived at the restaurant, he got out of the car easily on his own. None of us understood that, but for all of us, even for Carl, it was always a time of laughter, wonder, and joy.

A number of times the same quandary occurred, especially at breakfast times. His brain simply did not give him the signal it needed for seating himself. I realize now that his mind was not connecting with the presence of a chair, but at that time, I would become so impatient with him and with myself that I'd cry aloud. Amazingly crying can be a de-stressor.

Gradually, too, he found it harder and harder to know what to do to get himself out of bed. He was too heavy for me to pull into an upright position, although I would try by taking hold of both of his arms. Sometimes it took 20 minutes to get him out of bed. When he was finally up, I was emotionally and physically exhausted. Fortunately, I was never impatient about that. Surprisingly and at unexpected times, we become aware of the wellspring of kindness that is always available to us.

ACCEPTING WHO AND HOW WE ARE IS ESSENTIAL TO THE WELL-BEING OF ALL INVOLVED

To accept fully who we are may be one of a caregiver's bigger challenges. It took me awhile to discern deep-seated patterns that weren't necessarily compatible with what was happening to Carl.

I have a tendency to give my full attention to something that needs doing and to keep at it until it's done. This was always a part of who I am but it became more developed during years of meeting publishing deadlines. This meant that Carl was without my attention for hours at a time. He dealt with this by walking aimlessly around the house or sleeping in a chair. I often felt guilty about how

I was and at times altered my behavior but mostly I learned to accept what I couldn't change.

Another behavior, a more thoughtful one, that somehow balanced the one above, centered around meals. I was keenly aware of foods that Carl enjoyed and the ways in which he liked them prepared. I made at least one evening every week into a "culinary" event, and even when we watched the "Lehrer Report" while we ate, it was both a fun and comforting time.

While we were both writing, we used to go out to lunch at least once a week just to connect with each other. I continued doing that with Carl long after the onset of the disease. It was an unhurried time of being together; a time of communion. And, unlike other caregivers who have had experiences of resistance and bad behavior during similar outings, Carl seemed to need them.

Another less admirable way of being myself centers on taking walks. Carl always loved to walk and would go for a long one every day that he could. It was a way for him to exercise his hobby of taking pictures, kept him close to nature, and put his mind in a different channel than the work one. When he could no longer safely go for walks on his own I would take him but I would warn him before we left that I wanted to really walk which meant a fast pace. That meant I was walking ahead of him. He would often ask me to slow down a bit and I would but not for long.

In two instances while taking walks, I had started out at my own pace and he seemingly was following after. During one of those times I got way ahead but twice I looked back and he was behind me. The third time I looked back he was nowhere in sight. It frightened me. I quickly turned around and retraced the route but he was no longer on it. He also wasn't back at our house or on any of the nearby streets. By this time I was panicking. I thought of calling 911 but decided to call a friend. Since it was Saturday her son was also home so she said they would come right over with both cars so we could search in different directions. Amazingly, as I hung up the phone he walked into the house. I was so happy to see him that I didn't ask where he had walked. I still don't know.

I didn't learn from that experience and on a future walk I did as before – walked ahead at my own pace. In that instance he was trying to keep up with me and tripped. He fell face down and while trying to protect himself, scraped his hands and knees. He also had a gash over one of his eyebrows. This time when I turned around he was sprawled on the sidewalk, blood coming out of his wounds. I helped him up and took him to the house of a nearby neighbor. She helped me clean him up and put bandages on his cuts. There was so much blood that the cap he was wearing had to be thrown away. There were rips on the knees of his trousers and his hands looked like they had been in a fight. That was the last time that I walked ahead of him. From that day forward, we walked daily but we walked side-by-side. And, often, hand-in-hand. Regret over that still continues to haunt me at times.

There were other ways in which I had to reckon with the way I am and make adjustments. It isn't always easy to reconcile who we are with what it takes to be a caregiver. It's a continual learning experience—one that calls for a more loving and generous way of being ourselves.

ACCEPTING SUPPORT CAN MAKE A VITAL DIFFERENCE IN BOTH CAREGIVERS AND THEIR LOVED ONES

In hindsight, I know that I could have responded better to the many offers of support that I received and I strongly recommend being more receptive. Unfortunately, I thought that I could take care of Carl without much of the help I was offered and admittedly I managed pretty well. It's mysterious though, how much we can be controlled by wanting to "Go it alone" and wanting not to bother others. Another false and controlling premise is "I won't call on others until I really need them." I think I thought of the people who offered to be there for us as kind of like having an insurance policy – something to use when all other resources are depleted.

The people who knew us well didn't wait for us to call on them. In January of 2006, Carl was probably in the third stage of the disease and I was in full stage caregiving. During that month, a friend had completed 5 years as Country Director to the Peace Corps in Belize, CA. His home was near us. During his first visit to our home, following his retirement, he said to me, "Janaan, every Thursday evening from now on Blanca and I will bring appetizers and dinner and spend the evening with you and Carl."

I can't fully describe how important those evenings were. The night after the first Thursday that they were with us I had prepared dinner for Carl and me. After we were seated at the table, Carl looked around and asked, "Where is everybody?" I told him that our friends wouldn't be with us every night and that, for this evening, I was everybody.

On some of those Thursday evenings our godchildren joined us and gradually the evenings became a celebration of Carl. No one was in a hurry; all of us delighted in being together and Carl responded peacefully and joyfully to what was going on. Amazingly during those evenings, our love for him grew, and he reveled in the love that he felt from all of us. From that experience I realized that there is nothing more refreshing than what happens when someone is celebrated, not for what he or she was, but for whom he/she is right now.

This friend phoned every day and would often use the excuse, "I'm only ten minutes away and, if it's okay, I'll stop by." Those were grace-filled breaks and often those brief and caring visits made a saving difference, especially when I was having a harder than usual time.

Gradually I felt sure enough of his kindness that I'd call on him to sit with Carl when I had errands to run or appointments to keep. He didn't just sit with him. He took him for walks around the neighborhood and for scenic drives. On one of those drives, he took Carl to Mount Vernon, Virginia, and to Good Shepherd Parish where we had worked for 4 years with the Religious Education Committee. He was pleasantly surprised at how much of both places Carl remembered. What he did with Carl that day was a classic case of bringing into play memories that were still vitally alive in him and thereby, mysteriously, gave him a chance to realize that all of him was not gone. It's hard to describe, but when they returned Carl looked like a new man.

Three other friends didn't wait for us to ask for help. They would frequently call and invite us to their homes for dinner or brunch. These were always the best of times because Carl sensed how welcome he was, and that there were no expectations of him except to be whom and how he was. His diminishments didn't matter. Those were times, too, when I could let go and let be—real breaks for me as a caregiver.

Another long-time friend, a nurse, never tired of offering her support and was totally there for us during a time when I had to submit to surgery. Her genius was that she kept checking to find out what we needed and went out of her way to help. And, still, another friend would leave freshly baked muffins and other goodies at our door early in the morning on her way to work and I'd find them when I picked up our papers. She called daily to find out if we were okay and if we needed anything. And, she always reminded me that if I needed to talk she was there for me.

Another friend was an incredible help when we needed to access our Long Term Care Insurance. He contacted the company, got the forms, and literally filled them out for us. All I needed to do was sign my name. His support was invaluable when our situation was going through a radical change and I was almost crippled with panic.

One of our next-door neighbors offered to sit with Carl anytime I would need that kind of help. I didn't follow up on her offer but I always knew she was there if I needed her.

It's amazing to me now how many other people offered their support. The thing that I failed to realize was how serious these offers of support were. I hope that you, as caregiver, will be wiser than I was and will accept any and all offers of support. I've learned that to accept these offers is as much a gift to the giver as to the receiver.

RECKONING WITH LONELINESS DEEPENS WITHIN US THE VIRTUE OF HOPE

Loneliness was something that I had rarely experienced before Alzheimer's became a part of Carl's and my life. Most of the time, even then, it didn't last long because of friends who were frequently in and out of our home or who contacted us by phone and e-mail. I was also able to keep reading and writing, which kept me mentally and emotionally occupied. Then, too, Carl was a constant presence. He always wanted to be where he could see me so I was never alone. However, there were the in-between times in which friends, busyness, and Carl's physical presence were not enough.

The first time a wave of loneliness swept over me happened shortly after we were aware that Carl was experiencing dementia. I couldn't go to sleep one evening after we had had a session with his neurologist. All of a sudden, I began to cry. Somehow I knew our lives would never again be the same and the pain of that awareness overwhelmed me. And, even though Carl was asleep right beside me, I felt totally alone. To ease the emptiness, I began to pray the name, "Jesus" over and over and gradually I fell asleep. The next morning, I remembered clearly what had happened but the loneliness had passed.

Another time when loneliness seized me was in a restaurant that we often frequented. Carl opened the menu but he didn't have a clue what to do with it. I reached over and pointed to the entrée that he normally chose but he didn't understand. I went ahead and ordered it when the waiter came. I also gave the waiter my order but I was no longer hungry and I couldn't keep the tears from brimming in my eyes. I sensed it was another loss and it hurt mightily.

Loneliness, I've discovered, is both sneaky and unpredictable. Fortunately, in me, it's like a tide that goes in and out. The times when loneliness were truly like waves washing over me happened when Carl started to lose his train of thought every time he wanted to tell me something. In the wake of his inability to communicate, with words, I sensed something was happening in Carl that worked like an eraser. The thoughts he was having and needed to share were partially and sometimes wholly wiped away while he was desperately trying to form them. It was a loss of which he was acutely conscious and the loneliness I felt for both of us was unforgettable.

I learned, during those times, what a gift speech is and how precious it is to be able to talk to another. I was able to let go of the loneliness but I was never able to fully deal with the loss of that critical bridge that kept us meaningfully and lovingly connected. It's truly amazing how often two people, in our case, husband and wife, talk to each other. Because we were always working together on writing and speaking projects we were always talking about the content.

Another time when loneliness hit hard was after I'd put him to bed. I'd go to the living room to watch TV or to my office to do some work or try to do a cross-word puzzle. It would strike me how alone I was. It usually didn't keep me from doing what I had set out to do but the aloneness mitigated my enthusiasm.

Once in awhile my loneliness was tinged with fear. This happened a couple times when I'd wake up feeling ill. It was during those times that I realized if I were to have a heart attack or, for another reason would need help that I couldn't summon on my own, Carl wouldn't know what to do and even if I were to tell him what to do he wouldn't be able to follow the directions.

The loneliness I experienced during all the aforementioned times was nothing compared to what I experienced when I admitted Carl to a nursing home. I wasn't prepared for the loss of his physical presence. When he no longer was always where I was, I missed him so much that, at times, I could hardly breathe. At other times, I would sob and wail out of sheer grief. I dreaded going to bed because I missed cuddling up and lying next to him.

In that loneliness was the haunting question, "Will my life have meaning without Carl in it?" At first, no answer was forthcoming and I wept. Gradually, I adjusted to the emptiness and grew in the realization that while loneliness is a part of a caregiver's life, hope is also a part. With hope we can usually handle both the greater and lesser moments of being lonely.

THE LOSS OF DEPENDENCE ON ANOTHER AWAKENS POWERS TO COPE AND ADAPT

It amazes me how dependent Carl and I were on each other. I wasn't aware of this until Carl was unable to do things that he had always done. The first major sign of my dependence on him happened when I needed to change the thermostats on both our first and second floors. I read the directions. I thought I was following them as I made different adjustments. No change occurred! Carl had always adjusted them seemingly without a problem but when he wasn't able to do it, I had to seek outside help. I called the company that put the thermostats in. A technician came out and reset them and showed me what he did. All went well until they had to be changed again. Again I was unable to change them. I called the company again but told them that this time when the technician came he needed to bring simpler instruments. That solved the problem but at a considerable expense.

Another loss of dependence was connected to our computers. Carl wasn't necessarily a genius with them but whenever I ran into a problem, he was able to figure out what was going on and fix it. It never bothered him to have to stop what he was doing so that I could continue doing what I was doing. One day, he was unable to help me and I had to call a friend. He showed me what I needed to do if the problem were to occur again. I wrote the steps down so I wouldn't forget them. After the friend left, I felt keenly the loss of Carl as my on-site technician because I realized I had been robbed of a significant level of support.

The preparation of meals was another thing that we always did together, especially if we were having guests. Carl would set the table, take care of drinks, chop, stir, and wash or put into the dishwasher pans, dishes, and spoons when I was finished with them. It never seemed like all that much help until gradually he was unable to do any of it. The main fall-out of that loss was that we entertained less. That left me with a strange sense of isolation. I also felt kind of selfish about it because I knew that I could pick up the slack—I just didn't want to do by myself what we had always done together to prepare for guests.

The greatest loss of dependence came when he was no longer able to drive. It happened suddenly, as was the case with many of the other losses. We were on one of the local streets and without warning Carl started driving in the oncoming lane and it was with great difficulty and almost panic that I got him to return to the right lane. I had always depended on him to drive. He loved to drive and was able to find his way everywhere that we wanted to go. I just took his being our driver totally for granted. When I was forced to do all the driving it limited greatly where we went on our own. I had no trouble driving in Arlington but I no longer drove to many other parts of Virginia nor into the District or Maryland. Nor did we make longer trips like to Dubuque or to St. Louis to visit family. I grieved this loss more than any of the others but, as with the other losses, I learned how to deal with it. That's the mystery of the human spirit. The powers to cope and adapt are deeply embedded in us and new ways to compensate become available.

LAUGHTER ENERGIZES THE SPIRITS OF BOTH THE CAREGIVER AND THE RECEIVER OF CARE

Unexpected moments of delight and laughter are almost an everyday occurrence in a caregiver's journey with a person with Alzheimer's.

My husband, Carl, and I enjoyed many of those times. In retrospect, I know they made the journey easier. Some of these memories are etched in my spirit and I share them so that you may also become more attuned to them in your journey as a caregiver.

One day I thought Carl had forgotten my name, and I wanted to make sure that that wasn't happening. That evening at dinner I looked at him and asked him twice, "Carl, what's my name?" He looked at me with a bemused grin and queried in a mock serious tone, "Don't YOU know who YOU are?" We both laughed so hard that we could hardly stop. It was a wonderful moment.

Another instance when we both laughed aloud was when he was trying desperately to tell me something and I was trying as desperately to understand. He couldn't make what he wanted to say make sense so he stopped and in a complete and clear sentence said, "I know my life is impossible." As we laughed, we hugged each other, giving expression to the joy of that moment of lucidity and acceptance.

One of the funnier moments happened consistently. After he had had his hair cut and someone would remark about how good it looked, he would always answer, "I haven't seen it yet." Or, if someone would compliment him on something that he was wearing, he'd say with great seriousness, "I haven't seen it yet." And when we'd laugh at his response, he'd grin but probably not because he realized it was funny but because we were laughing. Somehow laughter eased and energized his spirit. It did the same to mine.

There were many more instances, but I'll share only two more. On the day that I admitted Carl to a nursing home, we were waiting at the Nurse's station. Carl noticed a gentleman having difficulty with something on his wheelchair. Carl walked over and helped him with it. Later that day, we met the gentleman again, and as Carl approached him he said, "I'm sorry I don't know who you are." Carl reached for his hand and said, "That's okay, I don't know who I am either."

Another memorable and funny moment happened one afternoon when an aide came into his room to take him to the bathroom. She asked, "Carl, do you want to go to the bathroom?" He answered, "Yes, next week!"

THE CONSTANT PRESENCE OF A LOVED ONE MAKES ALZHEIMER'S BEARABLE

As caregivers, we may think that getting away from the person is a way to become energized and refreshed. Oftentimes it can be, and sometimes it's necessary. What surprised me when Carl entered the last stage of the disease is how much he loved having me around. I could see it in his face. When I would tell him that I would be with him all afternoon (which I had the luxury of being able to do every day), a peace would settle over his face.

Even after he had lost most of his ability to converse, he thoroughly enjoyed having people around, and often I sensed, as did others, that he was in touch with what was going on. During his last months, when we had visitors, which blessedly were frequent, I would sit close to him and hold his hand which seemed to give him an anchor. Until his death in July 2007, he never tired of company, and toward the end the Hospice volunteers, sensing how much he appreciated their presence, lingered longer than they might have otherwise.

Presence, more than anything else, is the gift we, as caregivers, can give. Nurses, aides, and home health care givers provide physical care, but our loved ones are dependent on us for emotional and spiritual care. They need our presence as much as, perhaps, even more, than they need food and shelter.

I don't know the source of this quote, but I saw it on a bracelet: "When I don't know who I am, you're there to remind me." It exquisitely describes the presence we are as a caregiver to a person with Alzheimer's disease.

Resources

BOOKS

A Dignified Life: The Best Friends Approach to Alzheimer's Care—A Guide for Family Caregivers by Virginia Bell, MSW & David Troxel, MPH. (Demos Medical Publishing, Inc., 2005)

A Guide to Caring for People with Alzheimer's and Related Dementia: Caregiver Notebook. (Alzheimer's Association, 2009)

A Healing Journey: Coping With the Stress of Chronic, Life-Threatening Disease by Brenda L. Lyons, DNS, RN, FAAN. (Glaxo Wellcome Inc., 1998)

Alzheimer's Disease: The Dignity Within: A Handbook for Caregivers, Family, and Friends by Patricia R. Callone, Connie Kudlacek, Barbara C. Vasiloff, Janaan Manternach, Roger A. Brumback, MD. (Demos Medical Publishing, 2006)

Alzheimer's Disease: A Caregiver's Guide to Alzhemier's Disease: 300 Tips for Making Life Easier by Patricia R. Callone, Connie Kudlacek, Barbara C. Vasiloff, Janaan Manternach, Roger A. Brumback, MD. (Demos Medical Publishing, 2006)

Alzheimer's Disease by Paul Dash, MD, and Nicole Villemarette-Pittman, MD. (Health Communications, Inc., Health Professions Press, Inc., 2002)

Alzheimer's Disease: Unraveling the Mystery by the National Institute on Aging. (Alzheimer's Disease Education and Referral Center, 2008)

Ash Wednesday from Collected Poems by T.S. Eliot. (Faber and Faber Limited, 1993)

Beyond Forgetting Poetry and Prose About Alzheimer's Disease edited by Holly J. Hughes. (The Kent State University Press, 2009)

Caregiver Guide: Tips for Caregivers of People with Alzheimer's Disease. (From the National Institute on Aging, 2002)

Caregiving: The Spiritual Journey of Love, loss, and Renewal by Beth Witrogen McLeod. (John Wiley& Sons, Inc., 1999)

Caring for a Person with Alzheimer's Disease: Your Easy-to-Use Guide. (From the National Institute on Aging, 2009)

Coach Broyles Playbook for Alzheimer's Caregivers by Frank Broyles, 2006, www.Alzheimerplaybook.com

Dancing with Dementia: My Story of Living Positively with Dementia by Christine Bryden. (Jessica Kinglsey Publishers, London, 2005)

Dementia Care Mapping: Application Across Cultures, Edited by Anthea Innes, MSc, PhD. (Health Professions Press, 2003)

Family Therapy in Clinical Practice by Murray Bowen. (Jason Aronson, Inc., 1978)

Family Therapy Techniques by Salvador Minuchin and H. Charles Fishman. (Harvard University Press, 2004)

Hard Choices for Loving People by Hank Dunn. (www.hardchoices.com, Fifth edition)

Healing Arts Therapies and Person Centered Dementia Care, by Anthea Innes and Karen Hatfield. (Jessica Kinsley Publishers, 2002)

Help for Families of the Aging by Carol Spargo Pierskalla, PhD, and Jane Dewey Heald, MS. (Support Source, 1988)

I'm Still Here by John Zeisel, PhD. (Penguin Group, 2009)

Learning to Speak Alzheimer's A Groundbreaking Approach for Everyone Dealing with the Disease by Joanne Koenig Coste. (Houghton Mifflin Company, 2003)

Letters to a Young Poet by Ranier Marie Rilke. (Dover Publications, 2002)

Matters of the Mind and the Heart: Meeting the Challenges of Alzheimer's Care by Beverly L. Moore, RN, CS. (Strategic Book Publishing, 2009)

Memories in the Making® Creative Storytelling Through Art for People with Dementia by LaDoris "Sam" Heinly. (Alzheimer's Association, 2007)

On Grief and Grieving by Elizabeth Kubler Ross and David Kestler. (Scribner, 2005)

Person Centred Dementia Care by Dawn Brooker. (Jessica Kingsley Publishers, 2007)

Piaget and Knowledge by Hans Furth. (1969)

Psychology and Epistemology: Toward a Theory of Knowledge by Jean Piaget. (Hannondsword, Penguin, 1972)

Speaking Our Minds: Personal Reflections from Individuals with Alzheimer's by Lisa Snyder, LCSW. (W. H. Freeman and Company, 1999)

The Alzheimer's Action Plan by P. Murali Doraiswamy, MD and Lisa P. Gwyther, MSW. (St. Martin's Press Mew York 2008)

The Creative Age: Awakening Human Potential in the Second Half of Life by Gene D. Cohen, MD, PhD. (HarperCollins Publishers, 2001)

The End-of-Life Namaste Care Program for People with Dementia by Joyce Simard. (Health Professions Press, Inc., 2007)

The Enduring Self in People with Alzheimer's: Getting to the Heart of Individualized Care by Sam Fazio, PhD. (Health Professions Press, 2008)

The First Pressing Poetry of the Everyday by Donna Wahlert. (I Universe, 2003)

The Fearless Caregiver by Gary Barg. (Capital Books, Inc. 2001)

The Mature Mind: The Positive Power of the Aging Brain by Gene D. Cohen, MD, PhD. (Basic Books, 2005)

The 36-Hour Day by Nancy L. Mace, MA; Peter V. Rabins, MD, MPH. A Johns Hopkins Press Health Book. (Third Edition, 1999)

TimeSlips: Creative Storytelling With People With Dementia by Anne Davis Basting. (UWM—Milwaukee Center on Aging and Community, 2004)

ARTICLES

Barg, Gary, Editor-in-Chief, *Today's Caregiver—America's Magazine for Family & Professional Caregivers.* (2009 all issues)

Marson, D.C., Sawrie, S.M., Snyder, S., McInturff, B., Stalvey, T., Boothe, A., et al. (2000). *Assessing Financial Capacity in Patients with Alzheimer Disease. Archives of Neurology, 57,* 877–884.

McCawley, A-L., Telse, C., Wilson, J., Rosenman, L., & Setterlund, D. (2006). *Access to Assets: Older People with Impaired Capacity and Financial Abuse. Journal of Adult Protection, 8* (1), 20–32.

Moye, J., & Marson, D.C. (2007). *Assessment of Decision-making Capacity in Older Adults: An Emerging Area of Practice and Research. Journal of Gerontology, 62B* (1), 3–11.

Okonkwo, O.C., Wadley, V.G., Griffith, H.R., Belue, K., Lanza, S., Zamrini, E.Y., et al. (2008). *Awareness of Deficits in Financial Abilities in Patients with Mild Cognitive Impairment: Going Beyond Self-Informant Discrepancy. American Journal of Geriatric Psychiatry, 16* (8), 650–659.

Sherod, M.G., Griffith, H.R., Copeland, J., Belue, K., Krzywanski, S., Zamrini, E.Y., et al. (2009). *Neurocognitive Predictors of Financial Capacity Across the Dementia Spectrum: Normal Aging, Mild Cognitive Impairment, and Alzheimer's Disease. Journal of the International Neuropsychological Society, 15,* 258–267.

Tilse, C., Setterlund, D., Wilson, J., & Rosenman, L. (2005). *Minding the Money: A Growing Responsibility for Informal Carers. Ageing & Society, 25*, 215–227.

Triebel, K., Martin, R.G.H., Marceaux, J., Okonkwo, O., Harrell, L., et al. (2009). *Declining Financial Capacity in Mild Cognitive Impairment. Neurology, 73*, 928–934.

"2008 Alzheimer's Disease Facts and Figures," by Alzheimer's Association.

"2009 Alzheimer's Disease Facts and Figures," by Alzheimer's Association.

Index